Comparative Psychopathology

This book introduces readers to a more comprehensive and empirically based approach to psychopathology than any other approach in use by psychological professionals today. It incorporates all areas of psychological research, experimental and observation as well as clinical and medical. This approach presents a method that does not entirely replace methods like those in the DSM-5 but improves them.

Comparative psychology, the study of behavior across all species, has a solid place in this approach because it is where behaviors and psychological processes are studied in the most objective and empirically-sound manner. Areas covered throughout this text include not only the history of comparative psychopathology and comparative psychopathology as an approach to understanding psychological disorders, including anxiety and depressive disorders, better but also how comparative psychopathology can help advance psychology's understanding of terrible social ills, including poverty and violence.

By reading this text, readers will find essential information about how incorporating comparative psychology into understanding psychopathology can make that understanding stronger and how this approach can help psychology make for a truly better and just world.

Daniel Marston, Ph.D., ABPP, is a licensed clinical psychologist specializing in behavior therapy in the states of Pennsylvania and Ohio in the United States. He has two previous books and several articles published on the intersection of clinical psychology and behavior research. He also teaches statistics and research design in the Doctor of Education program at Liberty University.

Margaret Gopaul, Ph.D., MSCP, is a research scientist and professor holding a Ph.D. in clinical psychology with a specialization in neuropsychology, a post-doctorate in clinical psychopharmacology, and neurophysiology training in epilepsy from Yale University and the University of Connecticut (surgical neurophysiology). She is a research faculty at Yale University/ School of Medicine (Neurology) and serves as an associate research scientist at the Yale Comprehensive Epilepsy Center, and the Veterans Affairs Medical Center (Neurology).

Terry Maple, Ph.D., was an American behavioral research scientist, wildlife conservationist, professor emeritus (Georgia Institute of Technology), and zoo director emeritus. He was director and later president and CEO of Zoo Atlanta. Dr. Maple mentored 29 doctoral students at Emory University and Georgia Tech and wrote over 250 journal articles, chapters, and books on the behavior, conservation, and welfare of animals.

Comparative Psychopathology
Connecting Comparative and Clinical Psychology

Daniel Marston, Margaret Gopaul and Terry Maple

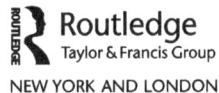
Routledge
Taylor & Francis Group

NEW YORK AND LONDON

Cover image: From The New York Public Library

First published 2025
by Routledge
4 Park Square, Milton Park, Abingdon, Oxon OX14 4RN

and by Routledge
605 Third Avenue, New York, NY 10158

Routledge is an imprint of the Taylor & Francis Group, an informa business

British Library Cataloguing-in-Publication Data
A catalogue record for this book is available from the British Library

Library of Congress Cataloging-in-Publication Data
Names: Maple, Terry L., author. | Marston, Daniel C., author. | Gopaul, Margaret, author.
Title: Comparative psychopathology : connecting comparative and clinical psychology / Terry Maple, Daniel Marston, Margaret Gopaul.
Description: Abingdon, Oxon ; New York, NY : Routledge, 2025. | Includes bibliographical references and index. |
Identifiers: LCCN 2024021823 | ISBN 9781032528816 (hbk) | ISBN 9781032503714 (pbk) | ISBN 9781003408918 (ebk)
Subjects: MESH: Mental Disorders--psychology | Psychopathology--methods Psychology, Comparative
Classification: LCC RC454 | NLM WM 140 | DDC 616.89--dc23/eng/20240614
LC record available at https://lccn.loc.gov/2024021823

ISBN: 978-1-032-52881-6 (hbk)
ISBN: 978-1-032-50371-4 (pbk)
ISBN: 978-1-003-40891-8 (ebk)

DOI: 10.4324/9781003408918

Typeset in Times New Roman
by SPi Technologies India Pvt Ltd (Straive)

Dr. Marston and Dr. GoPaul humbly dedicate this book to their esteemed co-author, the late Dr. Terry L. Maple. A pioneer in comparative psychology, Dr. Maple's visionary ideas paved the way for this book. These pages hold his last impartations to us and stands as a tribute to his brilliant mind and unwavering passion for knowledge. Dr. Marston and Dr. GoPaul are dedicated to upholding his enduring legacy through this work and book. Though Dr. Maple is no longer with us; his spirit and wisdom lives on through these pages. Rest In Peace, Terry.

Contents

Preface

In the vast expanse of psychology's terrain, the pursuit of unraveling the mysteries of the human mind and behavior is both timeless and imperative. It is within this dynamic landscape that "Comparative Psychopathology: Connecting Theory and Practice" emerges – a beacon illuminating the need for a paradigm shift in our approach to studying psychological disorders.

This book represents a departure from conventional methods, advocating for a broader perspective that transcends disciplinary boundaries. Grounded in the rich tradition of comparative psychology, it beckons us to explore the intricate tapestry of human and nonhuman animal behavior to uncover the underlying mechanisms of psychological disorders.

Our journey begins with an exploration of the foundational principles of comparative psychology and their relevance to the study of psychopathology. Through the lens of evolution, we delve into the origins of behavior, shedding light on how adaptive mechanisms have shaped the expression of psychological disorders across species.

As we navigate through the chapters of this book, we encounter a diverse array of topics – from anxiety and depression to addiction and trauma. Each chapter is meticulously crafted to blend theoretical insights with empirical evidence, offering readers a comprehensive understanding of the complexities inherent in psychological disorders.

Throughout these pages, we confront the consequences of marginalizing basic research in psychopathology and the subsequent loss of rich theoretical frameworks. Pioneers such as Darwin, Jung, and Skinner remind us of the integral role that basic and experimental research play in shaping our understanding of psychological disorders.

By integrating insights from diverse fields within psychology – including comparative psychology, behavioral neuroscience, evolutionary psychology, and clinical practice – this book challenges us to redefine our conceptualization of psychopathology. It urges us to embrace a more holistic understanding – one that transcends narrow diagnostic categories and encompasses the myriad factors that contribute to psychological well-being.

Furthermore, "Comparative Psychopathology" serves as a call to action – a call to transcend the limitations of traditional approaches and embrace a more inclusive and integrative perspective on mental health. It invites researchers, clinicians, and educators alike to join us in forging new pathways toward a deeper understanding of psychological disorders.

As we embark on this journey together, we extend our deepest gratitude to the scholars whose tireless efforts have paved the way for the insights presented in this book. We also extend our warmest welcome to the readers who accompany us, as together, we strive to illuminate the complexities of psychological disorders and pave the way for transformative advancements in mental health care.

Welcome to "Comparative Psychopathology: Connecting Theory and Practice." Together, let us embark on a journey of exploration, discovery, and transformation in the realm of psychological disorders.

Margaret Gopaul, Ph.D., MSCP

Introduction

Why We Wrote This Book

Chapter Material

This is a complex time for the field of psychology. With the vast number of clinical psychologists, clinical social workers, mental health counselors, marital and family therapists, and drug and alcohol counselors, there has never been a time with more mental health professionals around the world. These professionals have access to a large number of specialty fields, including forensic psychology, clinical psychology, counseling psychology, behavioral psychology, psychoanalysis, humanistic psychology, and many others. In this way, there have never been more opportunities for mental health professionals to be more specialized, if they prefer, or more informed across all areas if their goal is generalized practice.

Psychological research is also more substantial than it has ever been. There is more money spent on behavioral research than ever. More institutions than ever are involved in behavioral health research, allowing for much more representation in research. There are more academic and research publications than ever before. The advent of source open-source publications also means that there has never been more access to research for all professionals than ever before. Computer programs have also allowed for much more nuanced and focused research than ever before. Social media and technology have also allowed much more accurate representation than than ever for research samples.

Although psychology has never been so prominent throughout the world, it has never been so weak regarding its impact. Mental health problems are frequently referred to as different types of "mental health crises." There is little evidence that the vast amount of psychological research and psychological training has kept up with lessening the amount of mental health suffering that abounds throughout the world. At the same time, there has been this much psychological work there, and it seems there has never been this much psychological suffering.

DOI: 10.4324/9781003408918-1

When we wrote this book, the world just came through a terrible pandemic. Its impact is not over, and there is always the possibility that the pandemic could be back (also, when we write this, COVID cases are back on the rise along with other respiratory illnesses). There was a dramatic increase in the number of psychological disorders and psychological distress throughout the world, and psychological professions showed little evidence of being up for the challenge. When the human population across the world had to "shelter in place" for months, it led to dramatic emotional responses that impacted how people were able to function. This was especially the case with young people who lost a year or two of important socialization and learning opportunities.

Before the pandemic, it was not clear that mental health care was keeping pace with what was needed throughout the world. During and after the pandemic, evidence of the profession being unable to keep pace or effectively rise to the need that increases during crises was even more lacking. Other than the profession arguably doing well with rising to therapeutic needs associated with "social distancing" and increasing more ready access to what has become known as "video therapy," there was quite a lot missing in terms of the psychology field meeting the mental health challenges of the pandemic.

So, what happened? Why has a profession that has grown so large, in terms of number of professionals and amount of research and training work provided, done so poorly in meeting the world's needs? Why did the amount of what was available throughout the psychology field not keep pace with what the world needed?

We take the position that one of the answers to these questions is that the psychology field has become too territorial. There is too much separation between the different areas of the psychology field and not enough crossover. Although there is a great deal of research, training, education, and experience in each area, there is not enough collaboration between the different areas. This is exhibited between different areas of psychology not incorporating research from other areas, different professions not working with other professions, professional organizations and divisions of professional organizations not working with each other, and institutions not communicating with and working with other institutions.

There are many examples of this throughout the psychology field. Keep in mind that when we talk of the different areas of this field, we are referring to the different specialty areas (e.g., clinical psychology, experimental psychology, psychopharmacology, forensic psychology, community psychology, counseling psychology, etc.) and the different specializations (e.g., psychologist, clinical social worker, mental health counselor, psychiatry, drug, and alcohol counselor). In our opinion, each of these areas is represented so that their relevant professions and work are protected and supported but not so that there is much cooperation and crossover between them.

This lack of cooperation, collaboration, and crossover is evident throughout the different professional fields. Psychologists in the United States have the American Psychological Association, psychiatrists, the American Psychiatric Association (and, to a certain extent, the American Medical Association), mental health counselors, the American Counseling Association, and all the other professions have their own organizations. Different countries have their own versions of each of these organizations. Each organization stakes out its own position for its profession, but there is not much collaboration or cooperation between them.

Even when there are organizations with collaboration between the different professions, the territory is still being staked. In the United States, organizations for cognitive-behavior therapists allow members with different professional credentials (e.g., the National Association of Cognitive Behavioral Therapists) to stake out their own territory regarding the type of therapy and research their members emphasize. Psychoanalysis has been notorious for staking out territory for its training and research. Lawsuits and court cases occurred challenging rules set by psychoanalytic institutes on who can be allowed into their training and research programs (Cooper, 1990 & Lane, 2000).

Keeping focused on one profession also does not limit the impact of sectionalizing. One only has to attend a large professional conference to see the lack of cooperation between the different divisions within a profession. One example is the American Psychological Association (APA) annual conference. The association has 54 divisions, and each of them stake out their territory at the annual convention. An attendee will see a great deal of very important work presented and discussed throughout the divisions. Unfortunately, one will not see much crossover and collaboration between the divisions. Looking at the application forms to present, it is clear that collaboration is encouraged, but, in our opinion, as attendees at different conferences, it is not clear that it happens very much.

We are proud to say that not only does the approach to studying and understanding psychopathology here encourage collaboration, but its primary focus is on collaboration between fields represented by the largest APA divisions (i.e., clinical, and private practice fields) and the smallest (e.g., comparative psychology and quantitative research fields). It is also our opinion that it represents a field covered by a division in which two prominent names representing the extreme ends of the profession would have a home. Sigmund Freud and B.F. Skinner are two names often presented as the "polar opposites" of psychological theory. This may be simplistic, but they are often presented as the two main representatives of psychoanalysis and behavior therapy. They are then presented as the two opposite ends of psychological theory and practice.

Our approach in this book emphasizes comparative psychology research, and in the APA, comparative psychology is represented by Division 6. This division is called the division of "Comparative Psychology and Behavioral Neuroscience." Of all the divisions in APA, this one would welcome both Freud and Skinner. Freud was a clinician, but Skinner was mainly an academic, so the clinical divisions would be out—and Vice versa for the academic divisions. However, as a neurologist, Freud fit in with the Behavioral Neuroscience part of the division, and Skinner, as an academic who worked with animal behaviors, would have fit within the comparative psychology part. We find it rewarding and telling that our focus is one consistent with an area that would have the potential to bring together two of the opposite poles of our profession.

This book is about an approach to psychopathology that seeks to bring together all the main aspects of psychology. Comparative psychology is an area that emphasizes traditional research, and it is our position that it has a great deal to offer to the clinical field. Studying behaviors and psychological processes across species is at the heart of comparative psychology, and this is done through traditional experimentation and observational research like ethology. Comparative psychopathology, as we envision it, crosses over all areas of psychology and creates a truly comprehensive approach to studying, understanding, and treating psychological disorders.

We recognize that the separateness across different areas of psychology has not always been the norm. Freud was a clinician who also used the research approaches most used during his time. He also heavily incorporated research and writings by Darwin and his contemporaries in his work. Carl Jung did the same thing, except that his incorporation of animal behavior came from his personal experience growing up on a farm rather than psychological research. It is interesting that in his autobiography "*Memories, Dreams, Reflections*' Jung notes that one of the reasons his approach and Freud's differed in part because Jung, having grown up on a farm, had seen just how common some of the pathological behaviors Freud deemed as extreme (e.g., incest, patricide) were within the animal kingdom.

In its first half-century, psychology was much more replete with examples of clinicians and researchers whose work crossed over much more than would be common in the psychology field now. Names like Harlow, Maslow, Beck (Aaron), Ellis (Albert), Pavlov, and Watson are just some whose work in one field, clinical or research, crosses over into another. It is also the case that, although separateness currently limits much of the psychology field, crossover and collaboration exist in some areas and provide major advances. One prominent example is the work of Stephen Hayes and colleagues, who developed Acceptance and Commitment Therapy (ACT). Hayes started his work on Contextual Behavioral Science in behavior analysis work associated with research across animal species (comparative psychology) and moved this directly into work on effective psychotherapy approaches (clinical psychology).

In addition to acknowledging that we are certainly not the only ones trying to bring more collaboration into the psychology field, we also acknowledge that we are not the first authors to use the term "comparative psychopathology." That appears to be Howard Lidell, who used the term to describe the research work occurring on the "behavior farm" associated with Cornell University. Lidell was building on the work of Pavlov, who described the concept of "experimental psychosis" in his comparative psychology work. There was a reference to "comparative psychology and psychopathology" in an *American Journal of Psychology* article published in 1927 by GV Hamilton. Still, it does not seem the combination of the two words (resulting in the term "comparative psychology" being used).

Since Liddell, there have been different times when the term "comparative psychopathology" has been used in academic writings. A review of Google search using the term found articles referencing the term "comparative psychopathology" in 1961 and 1978.

Although we acknowledge that we are not the first authors to use the term "comparative psychopathology," we think we are the first to attempt a text defining the topic and clarifying what it offers to the whole psychology field. In many ways, our book is an expansion on an attempt to define the field comprehensively, started in an article called "Comparative Psychopathology," co-authored by one of our authors (Maple) in a special 2017 edition of the *International Journal of Comparative Psychology* on the topic of "Intersection of Comparative and Clinical Psychology," edited by another author of this book (Marston). Subsequent articles about this intersection have addressed how it could benefit all psychology fields, including an article by two authors of this book (GoPaul & Marston) on a recommended graduate course on the intersection of comparative and clinical psychology.

We are a mixed group of professionals writing this book. Two of us are primarily researchers and academics, while one is primarily a clinician. We all have academic appointments to range from adjunct professor to professor emeritus. Our specialties as a group include comparative psychology, behavior analysis, clinical psychology, forensic psychology, neuropsychology, cognitive-behavior psychotherapy, psychological assessment, experimental psychology, statistics, and clinical psychopharmacology. As a group, we have mentored many dissertation students and served as chairs of many dissertations and theses.

We all share a common dedication to making the field of psychology the best it can be. We seek to improve how psychology communicates among all its different areas and how research and experiences across all areas can make psychology strong and effective. If it is the case, as we believe it is, that psychology is not currently all the world needs, we sincerely hope that our work here helps move the field ahead.

References

Cooper, A. M. (1990). The future of psychoanalysis: Challenges and opportunities. *The Psychoanalytic Quarterly*, *59*(2), 177–196.

Lane, R. C. (2000). Psychoanalysis: The state of the profession. *Journal of Psychotherapy in Independent Practice*, *1*(1), 89–111.

1 Definition

Psychopathology from a Comparative Psychology Perspective

What "Comparative Psychology" Means

"Comparative Psychopathology" is an approach to understanding psychological disorders that incorporate behavioral research across animal species. This includes research on both human and nonhuman animals. It represents an expansion of psychopathology as it is primarily defined today. Incorporating the type of basic psychological and experimental research, as opposed to clinical research and diagnostic research, allows for more focus on the psychological constructs underlying psychological disorders.

What we seek in this book is not a new definition of psychopathology. We are looking for a more expansive one than is often used today and one that, in many ways, is the same definition used by the great minds of psychology from years past. In "The APA Dictionary of Psychology," the term "psychopathology" is "the scientific study of mental disorders, including their theoretical underpinnings, etiology, progression, symptomatology, diagnosis, and treatment" (VandenBos, 2007). This broad discipline draws on research from numerous areas, such as psychology, biochemistry, pharmacology, psychiatry, neurology, and endocrinology." Notice here how "psychology" is included but is not defined. Our view in this text is that the way "psychology" is incorporated in the modern understanding of psychopathology emphasizes only certain branches of psychology and leaves out others. Specifically, our view is that modern approaches to defining psychopathology focus only on the applied areas of psychology, clinical outcome studies, and research on specific diagnostic categories rather than on the basic and experimental research areas.

It is also our perspective that modern definitions of psychopathology have been limited in how behaviors and psychological processes are defined. Specifically, the focus has been only on these processes as they apply to humans. That certainly is understandable, psychological diagnoses apply primarily to humans. As of this writing, there is no structured method for defining psychopathology among nonhuman animals (an absence that we

DOI: 10.4324/9781003408918-2

certainly hope to help change). But even if the final product (e.g., diagnostic texts, assessment methods) applies only to humans limiting psychological research only to humans creates, in our opinions, serious barriers to fully understanding psychological processes.

Psychological research across species, the field known as "comparative psychology," offers ways of overcoming obstacles that research limited only to human animals presents (Papini, 2003). It is a major branch of psychology and is why we call our topic "Comparative Psychopathology." Research on nonhuman animals allows for natural observations across many different environments and in more circumstances than would be permitted in human research. It is also possible to control many more variables in nonhuman-animal research than in human-animal research. Variables impacting all areas of behaviors can be controlled when using nonhuman animals (e.g., where the subjects are raised and how much they eat every day of their lives) but cannot even be easily identified when using human subjects. In these ways, comparative psychology research is much more purely scientific (i.e., follows the scientific method in a much "purer" way) than is possible with human psychological research.

Comparative psychology research also allows for studying mechanisms of behaviors as they exist throughout nature. Psychological mechanisms like reinforcement, extinction, instincts, emotions, communication, and extracting information from the environment impact the daily functioning of all creatures. Understanding those mechanisms as they exist across species presents a unique way of comprehending how all beings function. If psychological functioning can be understood in ways beyond just what this means for humans, then psychology can indeed be understood as a science of behavior. Similarly, if psychological disorders can be understood in terms of how important psychological constructs impact their development and continuation beyond just for humans, then psychologists and other mental health practitioners can be said to truly understand these conditions.

Evidence of a Need for a New Way of Understanding Psychopathology

Comparative Psychopathology is an approach to understanding psychopathology that incorporates all of psychology. It emphasizes psychological research not just from the clinical and diagnostic areas but also from the basic and experimental areas. Its emphasis on comparative psychology also focuses on studies that address psychological functioning across all species. Comparative psychology is not the only branch of psychology that emphasizes basic and experimental research. Still, it is the one, as will be discussed later in the chapter, that has the most historical connection with understanding psychopathology. In the latter part of this chapter, we will make the case that incorporating comparative psychology into studying psychopathology is not a new way of viewing this field but is a return from how the field was approached for the vast majority of its history.

Before addressing the historical case for making comparative psychology a major part of understanding psychopathology let us look at the case that there a different approach to psychopathology, rather than just relying on the approach presently used, is needed. Presently, defining psychopathology centers around a text called the *Diagnostic and Statistical Manual* (American Psychiatric Association, 2013). It is presently in its fifth edition, called *DSM-5* (although it is likely that by the time this book is published, there will be a text revision called *DSM-5-TR*). We will discuss this text at length in different chapters of this book, but for now, our focus will be on what the text shows about what is emphasized currently across the mental health universe in terms of understanding psychopathology.

DSM-5 is a very large book (in print or online) that lists all the psychological disorders used by the profession. Its list has been deemed so comprehensive that most, if not all, major insurance companies use its disorders as a guide for determining what conditions they will cover (although this can become somewhat technical since they use *DSM-5* definitions of psychopathology because they match up with the codes of another list of all medical diagnoses called *ICD-10*). The *DSM-5* includes lists of criteria that are needed to define psychological disorders. So, for example, an anxiety disorder is defined by listing the anxiety symptoms the person has, how often the symptoms interfere with their functioning, how long they had the symptoms, and how to determine if the symptoms differ from symptoms associated with other disorders (used for the process of differential diagnosis). Clinical practitioners and researchers focused on defining diagnoses use the text to choose, based on the symptoms presented and whether all the criteria are met, the psychological disorder that best describes the individual or individuals with whom they are working.

Using the *DSM-5* for defining psychological disorders is considered a categorical approach that has limitations due to the "Yes/No" approach of whether a symptom is or is not present. This method has its limitations and could arguably be enhanced considerably or even replaced by a method that emphasizes dimensions of potential symptoms (thus called a "dimensional" approach) and the degree to which they are present or not. In a later chapter, we will discuss alternative diagnostic methods, focusing on one that fits particularly well in comparative psychopathology.

In this chapter, our focus is on what the *DSM-5* and its prominence in psychopathology says about the current state of this field. Since the *DSM-5* serves such a major role in the mental health field, looking at its limitations is a good starting place for looking at the limitations of how psychopathology is approached these days. It has been described as taking a purely descriptive approach rather than any sort of theoretical or research focus (Tsou, 2015). *DSM-5* is not the only place for defining psychopathology, but it is certainly one of the most important places.

DSM-5 is published by the American Psychiatric Association (APA), and that by itself is an indication of the role medicine plays in defining psychopathology these days. As different versions of the *DSM* were published, the dominance of the medical view of psychopathology became more and more evident (British Psychological Society, 2011; Musalek et al., 2010). There is even a term used at the time the *DSM-5* was being published to describe the dominance of this medical view; it is called the "medicalization" of psychological disorders (Pickersgill, 2014; Venkatesan & Suresh, 2023). Andreasen (2007) credited this approach of emphasizing the medical model of psychopathology with multiplying the "dehumanizing impact" of the *DSM* approach.

When looking at the medicalization of psychological disorders, the attention paid to only certain types of research is clear. Scientific accuracy is poor in many parts of the *DSM-5*, and this led to its developers seeing mental disorders as medical diseases (Lacasse, 2014). It is rife with scientific difficulties (Young, 2013), because of its focus primarily on medical research. This has led to the *DSM-5* and the field of psychopathology as a whole weighing heavily on research more important to medicine. Schultze-Lutter et al. (2018) summed this up as follows:

> In the wake of the immense technological advances, however, psychopathology has been increasingly marginalized by neurological, genetic, and neuropsychological research.

Critics of the *DSM* approach, which existed prior to *DSM-5* but certainly continued with this edition, have identified the limitation of an approach that leans so heavily on medical research. Andersson and Ghaderi (2006) summarized this approach's limitations for behavioral psychology practitioners and its limit on research relevant to behavioral psychologists. They called for an alternative method for diagnosing psychological disorders that rely more on a dimensional rather than categorical approach. In the chapter on diagnostic systems, we address such a method that fits well within comparative psychopathology.

The material presented here shows that the *DSM-5* has a real problem with a limited focus. Psychopathology has become focused primarily on definitions and research important for medicine. There is a need for a more expansive definition of psychopathology and a more expansive way of understanding psychopathology. This would be a view of the field that goes beyond medical research much more than is presently the case. Since psychology is the non-medical field most associated with research important for understanding psychopathology, this would be the field that needs more of a prominent role. But not just psychology relevant to clinical practice as that would be too close to what is already happening with medical research, as discussed earlier in this chapter.

What is needed today is an approach to understanding and defining psychopathology that incorporates all of psychology. This is where comparative psychopathology, emphasizing combining comparative psychology, comes in. Comparative psychology is likely the most comprehensive of all psychology's branches. It is comprehensive not only because it studies behaviors across all species but also because it is considered the study of all behaviors (Greenberg et al., 2004). Comparative psychology also crosses all barriers between different psychology branches and has connections with all those different branches (Marston & GoPaul, 2020).

Approaching psychopathology from a direction that incorporates all psychological science, not just that important to medicine and not just that from the applied and clinical directions, is supported by looking at the limitations of how psychopathology is presently defined. It is also seen in the difficulties with how psychology is understood these days. Misconceptions abound in how psychopathology and other psychology topics are understood. This is true of both students and professionals in the field and is often the result of a lack of incorporating comprehensive scientific findings that are presented about psychology (Dellantonio & Pastore, 2021).

Students, researchers, and practitioners as groups tend to show strong evidence of having misconceptions and misunderstandings of major psychological constructs. Research into this area has covered many different constructs, but depression is one of the most common areas studied. What tends to hold up an accurate understanding here is a lack of scientific understanding of the nature of depression (Sanz & García-Vera, 2017). One major misconception evident throughout depression research and education is that depression is caused primarily by the neurotransmitter Serotonin (Makovec, 2023). Note here how the misconception is due to a limited focus on one neurological explanation.

As shown earlier in this chapter, research important for medicine (e.g., neurological, genetic) abounds throughout the psychopathology field, and when psychological research is incorporated, it is typically clinical research. However, evidence shows that comprehensive psychological research, focused on helping advance scientifically correct explanations of psychological constructs, is most effective at reducing psychological misconceptions (Pieschl et al., 2021). Incorporating comprehensive research findings into fuller understandings of psychological disorders tends to help reduce misconceptions about those disorders, particularly when they are incorporated as a whole into what is presented, as this erases the time distance between when the student and practitioner learn the information and when they use the information (Kim & Kendeou, 2021; Lassonde et al., 2017). Incorporating all psychological research promptly, preferably with no delay between when all material about psychological constructs is presented and when the material is used, is essential, given research showing that readers of psychological material tend to hold onto their initial understanding of psychological constructs even after additional empirical research evidence is presented (LaCaille et al., 2019; Menz et al., 2021).

Research on psychology misconceptions supports the need for a comprehensive science of psychopathology that incorporates all fields of psychology. Comparative psychology, being a psychology branch connected to all other branches and studying all behaviors, is a strong candidate for what needs to be incorporated more into psychopathology study and understanding. This would be the best way for an approach to psychopathology that is indeed comprehensive and includes all research about psychological constructs.

Looking at where the field is in terms of limitations of *DSM* and the approach it takes to defining psychopathology shows the need for a different and more comprehensive approach to understanding psychopathology. Research on how misconceptions abound in understanding psychological constructs, particularly psychopathology, supports the need for a different approach that is more comprehensive. And then there is still one more area that shows the need for a different, more comprehensively scientific way of understanding psychopathology. This comes directly from the clinical side of the equation and starts with a discussion of what has been called "paint-by-numbers" psychotherapy (Silverman, 1996, 1999).

In the mid-1990s, Silverman (1996) introduced the term "paint-by-numbers" psychotherapy to stress the oversimplification of psychotherapy as evidenced particularly by the increased use of structured workbooks, worksheets, and other materials. "Paint-by-numbers" referred to a common way of painting appealing to a general audience where the individual would get a canvas with a picture drawn on it but to which color had not been applied. These painting kits included numbers on the drawings with colored paints with corresponding numbers. Individuals would use these kits to paint in the drawings by following which colors were supposed to go in which drawn areas. This allowed the person to have a feeling of creativity but only being creative on a superficial level.

Since Silverman first used the term "paint-by-numbers" psychotherapy, the use of structured workbooks and worksheets has increased considerably. This has increased emphasis on therapists and other mental health practitioners following pre-defined steps (Mariotti et al., 2022). What criticism Silverman lobbied against this approach initially has also been labeled the "manualization" of psychotherapy (Scaturo, 2001). There is considerable criticism of the increasing emphasis on using manuals in psychotherapy.

Criticisms have included psychotherapy being too rigid and structured, with no room for clinical experience or intuition, and harmful to the therapeutic relationship and alliance (Wislocki et al., 2023). Manuals negate the need for therapists to understand the constructs involved when psychotherapy interventions work and only require therapists to understand how to follow a specific set of steps (Galovski et al., 2020; Norcross & Lambert, 2019). Clinical expertise, which includes not only understanding "what" to do to treat psychological disorders but also "why" it works, has gotten lost in what current clinical fields emphasize.

Critics of manualization focus not only on the structured process but also on the research used to support this approach. Again, this is the clinical outcome research that typically involves comparing two or more groups, at least one of which has been given a certain treatment (Beutler 1998). This is known as "empirically supportive treatments" or "EST". Its prominence is evident because it is often considered the "gold standard" of how psychotherapy interventions are judged (Iliakis et al., 2019; Sakaluk et al., 2019). Criticism of this research targets not only the manualization limits summarized earlier but also how this research is based too much on patient self-reports and limits what other types of research are considered (Lampropoulos 2000). Another criticism of relying on clinical outcomes primarily for determining ESTs is the recent controversy of replicability in social science research (Sakaluk et al., 2019).

All this criticism of the modern approach to defining effective treatments for psychological disorders, which could be argued is a major facet in defining psychological disorders specifically and psychopathology generally, is a need for a different approach to showing treatment effectiveness. Kazdin (2007) and Nuttgens (2023) both present alternative approaches for identifying effective treatment approaches by emphasizing how change occurs rather than just whether change occurs. Kazdin presented considerable support that this is a much more effective and comprehensive way of determining that interventions are effective and leads to a more comprehensive understanding of psychological disorders (Kazdin, 2011). Nuttgens presents evidence that focusing on more comprehensive research for defining what is effective for psychotherapy can help to decrease the large number of treatments that all function the same way (what the author refer to as "Interventive Doppelgangers").

Throughout this section considerable evidence was presented that there is a need for a different approach to defining psychopathology. Emphasizing the *DSM* approach limits psychopathology to medicalized definitions. This approach also shows how present psychopathology emphasizes too much the "medicalization" of psychological disorders at the expense of other explanations. Neurology, genetics and biology become the only fields having a prominent say in how psychological disorders are defined. This also leads to a medicalization of how treatment is defined and emphasizes clinical out-come research. Taking this approach gives rise to misconceptions about psychological disorders that persist as more comprehensive scientific understanding is lacking. Psychopathology understood from this direction gives rise to an emphasis on psychotherapeutic interventions, negating any understanding of the "whys" of what treatments work at the expense of just the "whats" of what works.

As all this material shows, there is a need for a different approach to understanding psychopathology. This would be an approach that incorporates psychopathology research from all fields. It would be based on a comprehensive science that crosses over into all branches of understanding psychology. It would be a field that emphasizes all the factors that influence pathological behaviors (Scheveneels et al., 2016). In addition, it would be a field where all types of research methods, including experimental research, aim to elucidate the processes that contribute to the etiology, exacerbation, and maintenance of abnormal behaviors (Forsyth & Zvolensky, 2001). Psychological interventions based on this approach would focus not only on what approaches work but also on why they work.

Comparative psychopathology, an alternative approach to understanding psychopathology that incorporates comparative psychology more comprehensively, covers all these areas. It essentially "checks all the boxes" of what is needed for an alternative way of defining and understanding psychopathology and psychological disorders. Comparative psychopathology is also a field that has the added benefit of being comprehensive not only in how psychological disorders are understood but also in how information about psychological disorders is applied. Due to its focus on scientific study of psychological constructs across species, it offers material for defining and understanding psychological disorders in both human and nonhuman animals (Maple & Segura, 2017).

History of Comparative Psychology in Understanding Psychopathology

Throughout this text, we present an approach to incorporating comparative psychology research more fully into understanding psychopathology. Our position is that in recent decades, comparative psychology, along with other branches of psychology that emphasize basic and experimental research over clinical research, has largely been left out of the discussion of psychopathology. It did not used to be this way. Throughout much of the 20th century, comparative psychology and other branches of psychology served more prominent roles in how psychopathology and the treatment of psychopathology were understood.

Psychopathology as a field of study is traditionally thought to have started with the publication of Karl Jasper's book "Allgemeine Psychoatholgie" (In English, "General Psychopathology") in 1913. He endeavored here to develop for the first time a comprehensive work on the scientific study of psychopathology (*Stanford Encyclopedia of Philosophy*, 2023). Jasper based his approach to understanding psychopathology not just on major scientific works of the time but also on philosophical works. He also incorporated anthropology works and described one major aspect of psychopathology as understanding human life to be "inhabitant of an escapable form of danger" (Park, 2018). Although he did not specifically mention any comparative psychology work, his description of this danger can easily be seen as coinciding with the "flight or fight" responses that have made up so much of the discussion of anxiety disorders and similar psychological disorders over the past hundred or so years.

In the early 20th century, clinical psychology, which emphasized Freudian theory and the psychological constructs Freud and his contemporaries presented. Depression was described as "melancholy" (Akcan, 2005) and focused on the deep emotional impact of losses. As the 20th century moved on, a new approach that was more much based on academic work took hold. B.F. Skinner is probably the name most prominently associated with this movement as he worked heavily in academia but also wrote books that helped explain all human experiences using scientific psychology. This movement became known as the "behavioral psychology" movement in the clinical field. It was rather quickly incorporated by clinical psychologists who were looking at the impact of irrational thinking on psychological disorders. This incorporation of the two was called the "cognitive-behavior psychology" movement and it continued to dominate clinical fields for much of the latter part of the 20th century (Sampson, 1981). It is interesting to note that the combination of the two dominated even though some proponents of behavioral psychology, including Skinner himself, disagreed that this represented a different approach than behavioral psychology.

In the latter part of the 20th century clinical psychology started losing considerable ground to clinical psychiatry. Many different types of psychiatric medications came on the market and started showing considerable effectiveness. What this meant for the clinical field is that there was a preference for emphasizing medication as a treatment rather than psychotherapy. Medications were seen as working quicker and being cheaper than psychotherapy. There were attempts to show psychotherapy to be more effective over time and proponents here presented some evidence to support that a combination of psychotherapy and psychiatric medications is often the best approach to treating psychological disorders. But for the most part clinical psychology lost more and more ground to clinical psychiatry.

What was emphasized much more in earlier psychology that has become less much less emphasized in modern clinical psychology is an emphasis on all the scientific research conducted at that time. Psychoanalytic authors often used scientific findings not only from human psychology but also from non-human animal psychology. Freud emphasized a great deal of the work of Darwin and his contemporaries in his psychological theories. His work, in particular, shows the direct relationship between taking the scientific findings of the time and using those findings to present an understanding of psychological disorders. This certainly continued into the behavioral movement where B.F. Skinner did a great deal of his psychological work using research primarily on non-human animals. Skinner focused on the research for non-human animals and then used this as his explanations summarized in books and extensive papers on how psychological constructs observed in non-human animal behavior research applied to human behavioral psychology.

Psychological research, particularly that of the basic and experimental approaches, has also taken hey lower prominence in modern clinical definitions of psychopathology due to the rapid rise and significant rise of clinical psychiatry. *DSM-5* is a good example as even though it has emphasized a non-theoretical approach to defining psychopathology there is a great deal of criticism that it does emphasize a psychopharmacology model. This would be seen as another piece of evidence of the prominence of clinical psychiatry over clinical psychology when it comes to understanding psychopathology. When considering this issue, it is not irrelevant to consider that the DSM is published by the APA rather than any sort of psychological group.

What unfortunately happens when basic research is removed from having a prominent place in understanding psychopathology is that the psychological research underlying the theory also gets removed. Remember that early psychological theories were very much based not on clinical research but on the basic and experimental research prominent of the day. Darwin used what would be considered today to be ethological research and that played a large part in the Freudian theories (Serban, 1976). Carl Jung used much of his experiences observing animals on his farm growing up and his observations of psychotic patients on psychiatric units for his theories. He also pioneered "free association" not as a clinical technique, which it later became known for primarily, but as a way of gathering data for his theories. B.F. Skinner worked almost exclusively in the laboratory and used his experimental findings for his theories. His work kept clinical interventions to a minimum and the interventions emphasizing his work were based almost exclusively on psychological research findings (Schlinger Jr, 2011).

All this material is presented to make the case that the absence of theory in psychopathology definitions has led to an absence of the science that supported those theories. Basic and experimental research has been removed from psychopathology discussions in exchange for a focus on diagnostic and clinical outcome research. Defining psychological disorders in terms of what symptoms make up those disorders and how they differ from other disorders, the type of research emphasized in psychopathology definitions like that used in the DSM-5 provides only a limited understanding of the psychological constructs contributing to those disorders. There is an absence of understanding the psychological processes that lead to depression and anxiety, for example, at the expense of research that shows only what those conditions mean. Definitions are limited only to symptoms and the observable aspects of these conditions without a deep understanding of how these symptoms arise and what aspects of psychological processes contribute to their development and maintenance.

Incorporating Comparative Psychology More Fully into Psychopathology

Incorporating comparative psychology research, as is done in comparative psychopathology as discussed in this text, allows for more focus on the basic psychological processes contributing to psychological disorders. It allows for more consideration of not only what contributes to specific symptoms but also of what constitutes and maintains, for example, the "anxiety" part of "anxiety disorder." This means considering the role of the "fight-flight-freeze" response, positive and negative reinforcement, genetics, survival instincts, neurobiology, and habits in the development and maintenance of pathological anxiety.

Comparative psychopathology is an approach to psychological disorders that incorporates research not just focused on the disorders themselves. Diagnostic symptoms focus on the diagnoses and clinical research focuses on the interventions used to treat those diagnoses. Both are meaningful but do not tell the whole story. Comparative psychology research is the other end of the research spectrum. Since it focuses on nonhuman and human animals, it does not focus on research applied to diagnoses only involving humans. It incorporates research on the psychological constructs that underly the disorders. By focusing on the behavioral, neurological, genetic, environmental, and instinctual processes that cause anxiety, depression, psychotic, and other psychological disorders, comparative psychology presents a more comprehensive picture of psychological disorders than is presently the case with other approaches.

To fully incorporate comparative psychology into a discussion of psychopathology, it is important to define what definitions psychopathology has within comparative psychology. As with most areas of comparative psychology the definition of psychopathology addresses its role in both human and non-human animal functioning. Psychopathology has been studied throughout the history of comparative psychology and different aspects of the definition have been incorporated into the works of such authors as Darwin and Pavlov. These were some of the earliest authors discussing comparative psychology and it is useful to look at how they went about defining the term. We can then look at the end of this chapter about some ways that the term could be incorporated into an understanding of psychopathology that includes both comparative psychology and clinical psychology constructs.

When discussing any topic related to understanding human development and functioning from the perspective of psychology across species, the author with whom it is best to start is Charles Darwin. He had a strong interest in studying mental illness, and this led to his having an active discussion with the psychiatrist J. Crichton Browne (Gilman, 1979). Much of their conversations are contained in a set of over 40 letters that the two wrote to each other between May 1869 and December 1875 (Pearn, 2010). In these correspondences, we can see the most precise picture of how Darwin came to view the definition of psychopathology.

There had been writings on psychopathology earlier than Darwin that incorporated a contemporary understanding of human and nonhuman animal functioning. Most of these works incorporated the term "insane" to define people with psychopathology (a term presently used only in the legal field and referring to the most severe cases of psychopathology) and focused primarily on observable factors. These attempts to define and understand psychopathology gave considerable weight to facial expressions (Houston, 2003). Authors for whom this conceptual approach applies include Sir Charles Bell, Johann Kaspar Lavater, Christian Heinrich Spiess, and Erasmus Darwin (grandfather of Charles Darwin).

What Charles Darwin introduced into the concept of psychopathology was that psychological disorders could be changeable and even adaptable. He also presented in his letters the concept that psychological disorders could be adaptations to environmental factors (Alsawy et al., 2014). This idea that psychopathology was a changeable construct differed from earlier definitions, where it was seen more as a lifelong and permanent condition. It could be argued that Darwin's conceptual approach to psychopathology set the stage for later definitions promoting the idea that treating psychopathology is a much wider possibility than had previously been thought.

This idea that psychopathology could be adaptable and beneficial from an evolutionary standpoint also supports the idea that it could be present across all animal species. Troisi (2003) took a Darwinian approach to defining psychopathology and proposed that nonhuman primates could be seen as developing spontaneous psychopathology if psychopathology is seen from an evolutionary and adaptive perspective. When seen this way, terms like "depression" and "anxiety" could be used for both human and nonhuman primates. Key among this view of psychopathology is the idea that many types of psychological disorders may be rooted in some form of environmental adaption. If all animals seek survival and propagation of their species, then it is possible that psychological disorders may exist as an exaggeration of methods used for these goals. This key aspect of psychological disorders, primarily associated with Darwin's view of psychopathology, is one aspect that serves as the bridge between psychopathology being a construct used to describe both human and nonhuman animals. We will see more of this concept in chapters on social competition, depression, and "fight or flight" with anxiety.

Charles Darwin presented that psychological disorders could be adaptable. Ivan Pavlov, famous for his work on classical conditioning, took this further by proposing that psychological disorders could result from adaptive environmental responses. For Pavlov, neurosis was fundamentally a disruption in the normal equilibrium of excitation and inhibition processes within the brain's cortical tissues (Pavlov, 1934). He believed that excessive external stimuli or prolonged strains could disturb the balance between these processes, leading to abnormal behavior. If an organism, whether it is a dog (which Pavlov frequently studied) or a human, faced situations where strong, conflicting signals were present, it could lead to a breakdown in normal cortical function (Koch, 2019). Over time, these situations might induce what he described as "experimental neurosis" in subjects (Liddell, 1947).

Pavlov's understanding of neurosis was deeply rooted in his experimental findings and the framework of conditioned reflexes. He observed that when animals were placed under conditions of extreme and contradictory stimuli, they often exhibited signs of stress or breakdown, behaviorally analogous to neurotic symptoms in humans (Thomas & Dewald, 1977). For instance, if a dog was conditioned to associate a certain stimulus with food and then the same stimulus was presented without the reward or paired with a conflicting signal, the dog would show signs of distress and confusion. Pavlov believed that the pathological disturbances in the animals under such conditions were similar to neurotic patterns in humans. Thus, for Pavlov, neuroses were not just abstract psychological constructs but had a tangible, physiological basis tied to the brain's capacity to process and balance stimuli (Mineka & Kihlstrom, 1978).

Darwin and Pavlov presented a view of psychopathology that takes into account environmental factors and discusses primarily from the perspective of neurological impact (Paré, 1990). Darwin addresses more what would be later called the "frontal" areas of the brain. His work and the work of his contemporaries stress the impact of more advanced areas of the brain and discuss how pathology in human psychology sets people apart from how other humans appear and act. His work started with theories developed primarily from viewing photographs of humans with major pathology and discussing what likely led to those differences (Davidson, 2003). Pavlov and the work of his contemporaries focused more on what would be called the "lower" areas of the brain and discussed more the basic neurological areas that allowed human and nonhuman animals both to process and balance incoming sensory information.

It is interesting to consider that both Darwin and Pavlov have been connected in some important ways with the work of the most important clinical psychologists of their time, particularly Sigmund Freud. Pavlov's discussion of the experimental analysis has been compared to Freud's concept of the repetition neurosis (Dlin & Fischer, 1979). Their difference is that Freud saw sensory stimuli and environmental factors as tapping into unconscious drives that start a complex psychological response where the primary factors are not clear to the individual. Pavlov saw the processes underlying neurosis and other psychological disorders as primarily being an interaction between environmental and neurological factors where the primary goal is to reach a balance between organic functioning and feelings of well-being (Mowrer, 1939). An understanding of both environmental and neurological factors (including how the person responds to possible rewards and punishments, terms later prominent in the behavior therapy understanding of psychopathology) would be primary for understanding psychological disorders without the understanding of subjective internal drives.

Freud made several references to Darwin in his work and incorporated a good deal of his material and those of Darwin's contemporaries in his theories (Ritvo, 1974). Freud's theories of psychopathology are that he postulated detailed internal dynamics based in part on Darwin's theories that were based on observational and environmental studies. This is how Freud ended up with theories like the Oedipal complex, postulating a central incest sexual drive related to very early childhood experiences, when research based on observational data primarily (Morehead, 1999). It is interesting note that one of the major sources of later changes to Freud's theories is the recognition that Freud got much of what Darwin and his contemporaries concluded wrong (Ritvo, 1965). When attempting to formulate the specific internal factors that led to external behaviors (or covert behaviors that are made known through external behaviors like verbal statements) there often is a danger that a theorist will focus greatly on trying to guess what is going on inside the person and not giving enough attention and detailed consideration on what can be deemed from external observations.

Comparative psychology research presented in understanding psychological disorders early on in psychology's history presented material that was very useful for understanding what was observed and reported but not necessarily for understanding on a detailed level what was happening inside the individual. When all this is considered, it leads to a view of psychopathology focused on neurological structures and the environment. Learning and memory are given particular emphasis here. Psychological disorders are seen as conditions that develop in response to what the person learns and how they remember events in their lives. Comparative psychology offers more of a functional perspective of pathology where even behaviors deemed as "problems" serve some sort of function. Especially when seen from an evolutionary perspective, with a focus on adaption pathological symptoms, it can be theorized as being some attempt at adapting to environmental conditions. For example, troubling memories can be seen as a way of helping the person deal with traumatic events and remember them in ways that help the individual maintain some sense of self that feels manageable (Vanaken et al., 2021). Even if it becomes obvious to others that how a person handles their recall of a situation is not optimal, or even is clearly problematic, the individual may hesitate to confront that memory for fear of causing a major shift in how they define themselves. Focusing on how the person represents themselves would be seen as the language they have learned to explain to themselves and others who they are and their type of person. Notice how all this relates to neurological constructs like learning and memory and how the material lines up with psychological constructs like cognitive dissonance (Cooper, 2019).

What separates a comparative psychopathology approach from what could be termed a comparative neuropsychology approach (McNaughton & Corr, 2022) is focusing less on the neurological factors and more on how those neurological factors, like memory and learning, impact the person's functioning. Research most prominent in behavior therapy and cognitive therapy has been focused more on the pragmatic, where the focus is on understanding the function of behavioral and cognitive processing rather than a detailed analysis of what neurological areas are responsible for that processing (De Houwer, 2021). In the same way behavioral research, starting early on, moved away from discussing internal psychological processes (e.g., unconscious) as a means of defining psychopathology, they also moved away from defining psychopathology in terms of specific neurological factors (e.g., limbic system, amygdala). This latter approach was seen more as the realm of neuropsychology, which is often associated with different departments in the academic psychology realm, than clinical psychology (Hokkanen et al., 2020).

Reader's familiar with the history of clinical psychology will recognize issues brought up so far as ones reflected in the behavioral psychology movement and its understanding of psychopathology and clinical interventions. Most prominent in this field is B.F. Skinner arguably could be the researcher most associated with an intersection of clinical psychology and comparative psychology. His theories of pathology and clinical interventions were based largely on behavioral research with animals, primarily rats, and pigeons, and he saw the same constructs impacting nonhuman animals as impacting the development of psychological functioning in humans. His book *"Science and Human Behavior"* summarizes how human psychology can be understood from what is observed and does not need a detailed analysis of what is happening inside the individual to fully understand and address what is happening (Skinner, 1965). His work addressed the processes of learning and memory. Still, it did not give importance to trying to explain what internal mechanisms, whether they be unconscious psychodynamic processes or specific brain areas operating, were impacting those external processes. Skinner continued to speak against attempts to internalize psychological processes until the end of his career (Skinner, 2016).

Reviewing the works of Darwin, Pavlov, and Skinner in their historical context is important for this text because their work has primarily been seen in terms of its impact on clinical interventions. Behavioral processes studied by followers of these famous theorists have led to the development of three distinct phases or "waves" of behavior therapy (Hayes & Hofmann, 2021) over the past 70 years. These therapies are considered the most empirically supported therapy interventions (Huibers et al., 2021) used for major psychological disorders like depressive and anxiety disorders. Acceptance and Commitment Therapy (ACT) is based on behavioral psychology and was started based primarily on comparative behavioral research (Tarbox et al., 2020). Two major journals (Experimental Analysis of Behavior and Journal of Applied Behavior Analysis) are connected in terms of addressing behavioral processes across species and applying that research to behavioral interventions.

Considering that an application of comparative psychology research has been beneficial to the creation of a very influential behavioral application to clinical interventions for psychopathology, it is warranted to use this material to create a definition of the psychopathology being treated using these interventions. The material covered throughout this chapter shows that it would be a definition based on observable behavioral and environmental factors, even if the observable would require overt verbal statements reflecting the person's interpretation of internal factors. It would also be a definition focused on behavioral constructs but not focused on the other constructs considered more specific and detailed (e.g., unconscious processes, specific brain areas) for explaining those constructs. It would also define psychopathology as a behavioral process that occurs as the individual tries to adapt to their environment in ways that they perceive has some sort of functional purpose. Their interpretation may be wrong (i.e., their chose of how to reach the desired functional goal is not the most effective or beneficial) but it still comes out behaviorally as a way of reaching some desired goal. Using this definition would put an understanding of psychopathology on track to consistency with the theories underlying the behavioral therapy approaches effective with treatment and with the use of a diagnostic system like the RDoS later in this book.

Comparative Psychopathology Across Species

This chapter focused primarily on discussing comparative psychopathology as a method based on science for defining an understanding human psychology disorders. Although comparative psychopathology strongly emphasizes the study of psychological processes across species there has not been much discussion so far in this text about formal methods used to define psychological disorders in non-human animals.

There is simple reason why there has not been much discussion so far on methods used to formerly define psychological disorder in non-human animals, there is none. There have been attempts to develop systems of classifying animal behavior problems (including conferences as described in Mills, 1997). Still, these have been primarily systems based on specific disorders. One example is the system introduced for classifying separation-based disorders (De Assis et al., 2020). So far, there has been no one method of classifying all animal behavioral problems using one formal system.

Comparative psychopathology presents an opportunity to look at one system that could be used for diagnosing disorders across animal species (Boughton and Abramson, 2023). It would be wrong to say that the goal here is one system that is used for both human and nonhuman animals. Verbal communication serves a major role in human functioning but not in nonhuman functioning (Janoušek, 2019). As such, verbal communication and its impact would serve a major role in understanding human psychological disorders but not nonhuman behavioral disorders. This is one reason why the category of what would be considered veterinary psychiatry has been termed "veterinary behavioral medicine" (Sheppard & Mills, 2003). It is unlikely that one method of classifying and diagnosing behavioral or psychological disorders across species can be found but that does not mean that the same field can use research across species to understand both. That is what we will attempt to do with this text.

We propose with our discussion of comparative psychopathology to introduce a field that incorporates research across species to understand psychological disorders more fully across species. By using the term "psychological disorders" we mean conditions where there are differences in behavior, emotion and/or cognition that cause an individual to function differently from what is considered typical among their population. Our goal is to introduce a way of understanding these disorders beyond the current state that emphasizes research important for medicine and clinical outcomes similar to what is used for medicine. We propose a method that goes back to the origins of clinical psychology when all areas of psychological research were incorporated. This means to be a field of study emphasizing not only research on how these disorders can best be treated (e.g., clinical outcome research) but also basic and experimental research. Focusing on all research we propose will help the field of psychopathology get back to understanding not just the "what" symptoms are present and "what" interventions work but also the "why" those symptoms come to be and "why" those treatments work. We expect that emphasizing this knowledge comprehensively into an understanding psychological disorder will help all practitioners and researchers who try to help individuals, be they human or nonhuman animal, who suffer from those disorders.

References

Akcan, E. (2005). Melancholy and the other. *Cogito, 43*, 1–11.

Alsawy, S., Mansell, W., Carey, T. A., Tai, S. J., & McEvoy, P. (2014). Science and practice of CBT: A Perceptual Control Theory approach. *International Journal of Cognitive Therapy.* https://doi.org/10.1521/ijct.2014.7.4.334

American Psychiatric Association, D. S. M. T. F., & American Psychiatric Association. (2013). *Diagnostic and Statistical Manual of Mental Disorders: DSM-5* (Vol. 5, No. 5). Washington, DC: American Psychiatric Association.

Andersson, G., & Ghaderi, A. (2006). Overview and analysis of the behaviourist criticism of the Diagnostic and Statistical Manual of Mental Disorders (DSM). *Clinical Psychologist, 10*(2), 67–77.

Andreasen, N. C. (2007). DSM and the death of phenomenology in America: An example of unintended consequences. *Schizophrenia Bulletin, 33*, 108–112. 10.1093/schbul/sbl054.

Beutler, L. E. (1998). Identifying empirically supported treatments: What if we didn't? *Journal of Consulting and Clinical Psychology, 66*(1), 113–120. https://doi.org/10.1037/0022006X.66.1.113

Boughton, B. A., & Abramson, C. I. (2023). The role of comparative psychology in the training of veterinarians. *Animals, 13*(14), 2315.

British Psychological Society. (2011). Response to American Psychiatric Association: DSM-5 Development. http://apps.bps.org.uk/_publicationfiles/consultation-responses/DSM-5%202011%20-%20BPS%20response.pdf

Cooper, J. (2019). Cognitive dissonance: Where we've been and where we're going. *International Review of Social Psychology, 32*(1), 7.

Davidson, R. J. (2003). Darwin and the neural bases of emotion and affective style. *Annals of the New York Academy of Sciences, 1000*(1), 316–336.

De Assis, L. S., Matos, R., Pike, T. W., Burman, O. H., & Mills, D. S. (2020). Developing diagnostic frameworks in veterinary behavioral medicine: Disambiguating separation related problems in dogs. *Frontiers in Veterinary Science, 6*, 499.

De Houwer, J. (2021). On the challenges of cognitive psychopathology research and possible ways forward: Arguments for a pragmatic cognitive approach. *Current Opinion in Psychology, 41*, 96–99.

Dellantonio, S., & Pastore, L. (2021). Ignorance, misconceptions and critical thinking. *Synthese, 198*(8), 7473–7501.

Dlin, B. M., & Fischer, H. K. (1979). The anniversary reaction: A meeting of Freud and Pavlov. *Psychosomatics, 20*(11), 749–755.

Forsyth, J. P., & Zvolensky, M. J. (2001). Experimental psychopathology, clinical science, and practice: An irrelevant or indispensable alliance? *Applied and Preventive Psychology, 10*(4), 243–264.

Galovski, T. E., Nixon, R. D., & Kaysen, D. (2020). *Flexible Applications of Cognitive Processing Therapy: Evidence-Based Treatment Methods*. Academic Press.

Gilman, S. L. (1979). Darwin sees the insane. *Journal of the History of the Behavioral Sciences*, *15*(3), 253–262.

Greenberg, G., Partridge, T., Weiss, E., & Pisula, W. (2004). Comparative psychology, a new perspective for the 21st century: Up the spiral staircase. *Developmental Psychobiology: The Journal of the International Society for Developmental Psychobiology*, *44*(1), 1–15.

Hayes, S. C., & Hofmann, S. G. (2021). "Third-wave" cognitive and behavioral therapies and the emergence of a process-based approach to intervention in psychiatry. *World Psychiatry*, *20*(3), 363–375.

Hokkanen, L., Barbosa, F., Ponchel, A., Constantinou, M., Kosmidis, M. H., Varako, N. & Hessen, E. (2020). Clinical neuropsychology as a specialist profession in European health care: Developing a benchmark for training standards and competencies using the Europsy Model?. *Frontiers in Psychology*, *11*, 559134.

Houston, R. A. (2003). The face of madness in eighteenth-and early nineteenth-century Scotland. *Eighteenth-Century Life*, *27*(2), 49–66.

Huibers, M. J., Lorenzo-Luaces, L., Cuijpers, P., & Kazantzis, N. (2021). On the road to personalized psychotherapy: A research agenda based on cognitive behavior therapy for depression. *Frontiers in Psychiatry*, *11*, 607508.

Iliakis, E. A., Sonley, A. K., Ilagan, G. S., & Choi-Kain, L. W. (2019). Treatment of borderline personality disorder: Is supply adequate to meet public health needs?. *Psychiatric Services*, *70*(9), 772–781.

Janoušek, J. (2019). Verbal Communication as a Psychological Problem. *Journal of Russian & East European Psychology*, *56*(1), 1–85.

Kazdin, A. E. (2007). Mediators and mechanisms of change in psychotherapy research. *Annual Review of Clinical Psychology*, *3*, 1–27.

Kazdin, A. E. (2011). Evidence-based treatment research: Advances, limitations, and next steps. *American Psychologist*, *66*(8), 685–698. https://doi.org/10.1037/a0024975

Kim, J., & Kendeou, P. (2021). Knowledge transfer in the context of refutation texts. *Contemporary Educational Psychology*, *67*, 102002.

Koch, U. (2019). The uses of trauma in experiment: Traumatic stress and the history of experimental neurosis, c. 1925–1975. *Science in Context*, *32*(3), 327–351.

LaCaille, R. A., LaCaille, L. J., Damsgard, E., & Maslowski, A. K. (2019). Refuting mental health misconceptions: A quasi-experiment with abnormal psychology courses. *Psychology Learning & Teaching*, *18*(3), 275–289.

Lacasse, J. R. (2014). After DSM-5: A critical mental health research agenda for the 21st century. *Research on Social Work Practice*, *24*(1), 5–10.

Lampropoulos, G. K. (2000). A reexamination of the empirically supported treatments critiques. *Psychotherapy Research*, *10*(4), 474–487, DOI:10.1093/ptr/10.4.474

Lassonde, K. A., Kolquist, M., & Vergin, M. (2017). Revising psychology misconceptions by integrating a refutation-style text framework into poster presentations. *Teaching of Psychology*, *44*(3), 255–262.

Liddell, H. S. (1947). The experimental neurosis. *Annual Review of Physiology*, *9*(1), 569–580.

Makovec, T. (2023). Serotonin and Depression. A Sceptical Eye's View. *Journal of Biomedical Research and Environmental Sciences*, *2766*, 2276.

Maple, T. L., & Segura, V. D. (2017). Comparative psychopathology: Connecting comparative and clinical psychology. *International Journal of Comparative Psychology*, *30*.

Mariotti, M., Saba, G., & Stratton, P. (2022). Towards a truly systemic account of the current and future of manualisation. In: *Handbook of Systemic Approaches to Psychotherapy Manuals: Integrating Research, Practice, and Training* (pp. 1–12). Cham: Springer International Publishing.

Marston, D. & Gopaul, M. T. (2020). Considerations for an integrated undergraduate comparative and clinical psychology course. *International Journal of Comparative Psychology*, *33*. Available online: https://escholarship.org/uc/item/41j4c087 (accessed on 1 December 2023).

McNaughton, N., & Corr, P. J. (2022). The non-human perspective on the neurobiology of temperament, personality, and psychopathology: What's next?. *Current Opinion in Behavioral Sciences*, *43*, 255–262.

Menz, C., Spinath, B., Hendriks, F., & Seifried, E. (2021). Reducing educational psychological misconceptions: How effective are standard lectures, refutation lectures, and instruction in information evaluation strategies? *Scholarship of Teaching and Learning in Psychology*.

Mills, D. S. (1997). Conceptualizing behaviour problems-separating a dog's bite from its owner's problem. In: *Proceedings of the first International Conference on Veterinary Behavioural Medicine*. Birmingham: Universities Federation for Animal Welfare.

Mineka, S., & Kihlstrom, J. F. (1978). Unpredictable and uncontrollable events: A new perspective on experimental neurosis. *Journal of Abnormal Psychology*, *87*(2), 256262.

Morehead, D. (1999). Oedipus, Darwin, and Freud: One big, happy family?. *The Psychoanalytic Quarterly*, *68*(3), 347–375.

Mowrer, O. H. (1939). A stimulus-response analysis of anxiety and its role as a reinforcing agent. *Psychological Review*, *46*(6), 553–565. https://doi.org/10.1037/h0054288

Musalek, M., Larach-Walters, V., Lepine, J. P., Millet, B., Gaebel, W., & on behalf of the WSFSBP Task Force on Nosology and Psychopathology. (2010). Psychopathology in the 21st century. *The World Journal of Biological Psychiatry* *11*, 844–851. 10.3109/15622975.2010.510207

Norcross, J. C., & Lambert, M. J. (2019). Evidence-based psychotherapy relationships: The third task force. *Psychotherapy Relationships that Work*, *1*, 1–23.

Nuttgens, S. (2023). Of interventive doppelgangers and other barriers to evidence-based practice in psychotherapy. *Journal of Psychotherapy Integration*, *33*(1), 233–246.

Papini, M. R. (2003). Comparative psychology. *Handbook of Research Methods in Experimental Psychology*, 211–240.

Paré, W. P. (1990). Pavlov as a psychophysiological scientist. *Brain Research Bulletin*, *24*(5), 643–649.

Park, S. C. (2018). Karl Jaspers' general psychopathology (Allgemeine Psychopathologie) and its implication for the current psychiatry. *Psychiatry Investigation*, *16*(2), 99–108. doi:10.30773/pi.2018.12.19.2. Epub 2019 Feb 21. Erratum in: Psychiatry Investig. 2020 Feb;17(2):177. PMID: 30808115; PMCID: PMC6393754.

Pavlov, I. P. (1934). An attempt at a physiological interpretation of obsessional neurosis and paranoia. *Journal of Mental Science*, *80*(329), 187–197.

Pearn, A. M. (2010). 'This excellent observer …': The correspondence between Charles Darwin and James Crichton-Browne, 1869–75. *History of Psychiatry*, *21*(2), 160–175. doi:10.1177/0957154X10363961

Pickersgill, M. D. (2014). Debating DSM-5: diagnosis and the sociology of critique. *Journal of Medical Ethics*, *40*(8), 521–525.

Pieschl, S., Budd, J., Thomm, E., & Archer, J. (2021). Effects of raising student teachers' metacognitive awareness of their educational psychological misconceptions. *Psychology Learning & Teaching, 20*(2), 214–235.

Ritvo, L. B. (1965). Darwin as the source of Freud's neo-Lamarckianism. *Journal of the American Psychoanalytic Association, 13*(3), 499–517.

Ritvo, L. B. (1974). The impact of Darwin on Freud. *The Psychoanalytic Quarterly, 43*(2), 177–192.

Sakaluk, J. K., Williams, A. J., Kilshaw, R. E., & Rhyner, K. T. (2019). Evaluating the evidential value of empirically supported psychological treatments (ESTs): A meta-scientific review. *Journal of Abnormal Psychology, 128*(6), 500–509. https://doi.org/10.1037/abn0000421

Sampson, E. E. (1981). Cognitive psychology as ideology. *American Psychologist, 36*(7), 730–743. https://doi.org/10.1037/0003-066X.36.7.730

Sanz, J., & García-Vera, M. P. (2017). Misconceptions about depression and its treatment (I). *Papeles del Psicólogo., 38*(3), 169–176.

Scaturo, D. J. (2001). The evolution of psychotherapy and the concept of manualization: An integrative perspective. *Professional Psychology: Research and Practice, 32*(5), 522–530. https://doi.org/10.1037/0735-7028.32.5.522

Scheveneels, S., Boddez, Y., Vervliet, B., & Hermans, D. (2016). The validity of laboratory-based treatment research: Bridging the gap between fear extinction and exposure treatment. *Behaviour Research and Therapy, 86*, 87–94.

Schlinger Jr, H. D. (2011). Skinner as missionary and prophet: A review of Burrhus F. Skinner: Shaper of Behaviour. *Journal of Applied Behavior Analysis, 44*(1), 217–225.

Schultze-Lutter, F., Schmidt, S. J., & Theodoridou, A. (2018). Psychopathology—a precision tool in need of re-sharpening. *Frontiers in Psychiatry, 9*, 446.

Serban, G. (1976). The significance of ethology for psychiatry. In: *Animal Models in Human Psychobiology* (pp. 279–289). Boston, MA: Springer US.

Sheppard, G., & Mills, D. S. (2003). Construct models in veterinary behavioural medicine: Lessons from the human experience. *Veterinary Research Communications, 27*, 175–191.

Silverman, W. H. (1996). Cookbooks, manuals, and paint-by-numbers: Psychotherapy in the 90's. *Psychotherapy: Theory, Research, Practice, Training, 33*(2), 207.

Silverman, W. H. (1999). Editorial: If it's Tuesday with depressive symptoms it must be cognitive-behavior therapy. *Psychotherapy: Theory, Research, Practice, Training, 36*(4), 317–319. https://doi.org/10.1037/h0092419

Skinner, B. F. (1965). *Science and Human Behavior.* No. 92904. Simon and Schuster.

Skinner, B. F. (2016). Why I am not a cognitive psychologist. In: *Approaches to Cognition* (pp. 79–90). Routledge.

Stanford Encyclopedia of Philosophy. (2023). *"Karl Jaspers".* Available at https://plato.stanford.edu/entries/jaspers/. Accessed December 5, 2023.

Tarbox, J., Szabo, T. G., & Aclan, M. (2020). Acceptance and commitment training within the scope of practice of applied behavior analysis. *Behavior Analysis and Practice, 15*(1), 11–32. doi:10.1007/s40617-020-00466-3. PMID: 35340381; PMCID: PMC8854459.

Thomas, E., & DeWald, L. (1977). Neurosis: experimental neurosis: neuropsychological analysis. In: J. D. Maser & M. E. P. Seligman (Eds.), *Psychopathology: Experimental models* (pp. 214–231). W H Freeman/Times Books/Henry Holt & Co.

Troisi, A. (2003). Psychopathology. In: D. Maestripieri (Ed.), *Primate Psychology* (pp. 451–470). Harvard University Press.

Tsou, J. Y. (2015). DSM-5 and psychiatry's second revolution: Descriptive vs. theoretical approaches to psychiatric classification. *The DSM-5 in Perspective: Philosophical Reflections on the Psychiatric Babel*, 43–62.

Vanaken, L., Boddez, Y., Bijttebier, P., & Hermans, D. (2021). Reasons to remember: A functionalist view on the relation between memory and psychopathology. *Current Opinion in Psychology*, *41*, 88–95.

VandenBos, G. R. (Ed.). (2007). *APA Dictionary of Psychology*. American Psychological Association.

Venkatesan, S., & Suresh, A. (2023). Critique of DSM, medicalization and graphic medicine. *Journal of Graphic Novels and Comics*, *14*(2), 233–247.

Wislocki, K., Tran, M. L., Petti, E., Hernandez-Ramos, R., Cenkner, D., Bridgwater, M., Naderi, G., Walker, L., & Zalta, A.K. (2023). The past, present, and future of psychotherapy manuals: protocol for a scoping review. *JMIR Research Protocols*, *30*(12), e47708. doi:10.2196/47708. PMID: 37389903; PMCID: PMC10365618.

Young, G. (2013). Breaking bad: DSM-5 description, criticisms, and recommendations. *Psychological Injury and Law*, *6*, 345–348. https://doi.org/10.1007/s12207-013-9181-8

2 Comparative Psychopathology and Diagnostic Systems

Introduction

Comparative psychopathology addresses how psychological disorders are interpreted from a base of empirical research findings. Behavioral research across species has shown considerable evidence of what factors impact how individuals function. This includes behavioral, cognitive, and emotional functioning and allows for understanding functioning in all human and nonhuman animals. It allows for an understanding of psychopathology as defined not only by what symptoms are observed but also by what research shows about how those symptoms are created and maintained.

What this chapter addresses is how comparative psychopathology can best be conceptualized from a diagnostic system. Clinicians use diagnostic systems to help define the disorders they treat and for guidance on how best to talk about, understand, and intervene in psychological disorders. It is not likely that any comprehensive approach to understanding psychopathology, like the one discussed throughout this book, can exist without having some sort of formal diagnostic system. That is why this chapter focuses on the diagnostic system that fits best within a comparative psychopathology framework.

Diagnostic Systems

Clinicians and researchers discuss clinical disorders and need a common language for how they discuss disorders. They need a common language for how they communicate about psychological disorders. If clinicians and researchers are going to talk, for example, about understanding and treating conditions where the person has a lasting sense of hopelessness and helplessness along with constant sadness and lack of energy and motivation they need a diagnostic classification for depression. If clinicians and researchers are going to discuss clinical conditions where patients see things that are not there, hear things that are not there, react in bizarre ways to other people,

DOI: 10.4324/9781003408918-3

and have an inability to care for themselves adequately then they must be able to discuss schizophrenia.

This common language about clinical psychological disorders requires not only common terms but also common ways those terms are defined. Diagnostic classification systems are how psychopathology terms are identified and defined. At the very least these systems provide specific behaviors and other symptoms that are associated with the psychological disorders. There is also information provided that helps to distinguish one disorder from another. Psychological disorders often share symptoms with other disorders so being able to identify what distinguishes the disorders from each other is essential.

What is often missing from diagnostic systems is a connection to research beyond just research on the symptoms associated with clinical disorders. Broader psychological research about major psychological constructs, processes by which behavioral, cognitive, and affective systems function and system interactions is often missing from diagnostic systems. Leaving out this material leads out important information essential for understanding possible causes and conceptualizing clinical cases. Diagnostic systems allow for common definitions of psychological disorders but do not always provide information about how to conceptualize why those disorders exist and how they are maintained. Having this information allows clinicians and researchers alike to enter into situations where the diagnostic terminology is used with not only an understanding of what the terminology means but also how the conditions being defined came about. This allows for more informed decisions regarding treatment and investigation.

Diagnostic systems that leave out material for case conceptualization led to those systems failing to achieve their full purpose (Hayes et al., 2020). These systems did not always work that way. Different attempts at diagnostic systems for psychological professionals started being used widely in the 1950s. Once they started being used there were different attempts to try and make them more effective. When diagnostic systems were in those stages of development there was more of a focus on material used for not only defining clinical disorders but also for case conceptualization and treatment decisions.

It is in this area where the most common diagnostic system used by clinicians is lacking. The Diagnostic and Statistical Manual, now in its fifth edition, or the "DSM-5" (American Psychiatric Association, 2013) is a system focused primarily on categorization rather than conceptualization. It is used by clinicians and researchers around the world to diagnose and study mental disorders. Although it is accepted widely as the "final word" in diagnoses its development has been mired in many different political and professional controversies (Shorter, 2022). These controversies led to the DSM being very limited in what material could be agreed on among all the different individuals and professional groups involved with its development. Despite its wide use, it has been criticized for being limited for clinicians due to it providing very little direction for case conceptualization.

Clinicians and researchers in the United States primarily use the DSM-5 diagnostic system but it is not the only system. In Europe, the most common diagnostic system is the International Classification of Disease, now in its 11th edition (ICD-11). This system focuses on definitions but does not list criteria in the same way as DSM-5. Much like DSM-5 the ICD-11 focuses on self-reported or clinically observable symptoms and purposely stays away from theories or causes (Gaebel et al., 2020). Because both the DSM-5 and ICD-11 are used so prominently across the world there are attempts to try and harmonize the two systems (First et al., 2021).

What both the DSM-5 and ICD-11 have in common is their atheoretical base. Authors of both systems worked to make sure both systems are devoid of stressing any one theoretical school related to psychopathology. There is not supposed to be any preference given to any one direction in terms of deciding how psychological disorders develop. This is supposed to be the case although DSM-5 has been shown a preference for neurological explanations (Lasalvia, 2015).

Alternative systems to the DSM-5 and ICD-11 are often presented as additions to these descriptive systems rather than replacements. One that has received the most attention is the Psychodynamics Diagnostic Manual or "PDM" (PDM Task Force, 2006). This manual, currently in its second edition, focuses on a dimensional system. Rather than look at disorders in a "Yes" or "No" system in terms of whether symptoms are present or not, the PDM focuses on dimensions of different personality constructs and identifies where the individual falls on each dimension (Lingiardi et al., 2015). Practitioners using the PDM continue to use disorder terminology from the DSM-5 but use the PDM as a way of giving more depth to describe symptomology. Since this method is anchored in a theoretical school, it also allows practitioners more room to consider psychodynamic research when making diagnostic decisions.

Research Domain Criteria (RDoC)

When considering a diagnostic system that fits within the field of comparative psychopathology, a dimensional system like the PDM would fit well. As with the PDM, this could make it a complement to the DSM in providing a more complex way to define psychopathology. Comparative psychology is a field much more solidly based on traditional research than the PDM, whose basis is in the psychodynamic and psychoanalytic literature, so the focus would need to be more in that direction. Theoretical constructs could still play a role, but the focus would have to be on constructs consistent with empirical research findings. If there had to be a theoretical school identified for the system that works best for comparative psychopathology it would likely be applied behavior analysis.

Enter the Research Domain Criteria or "RDoC" (Casey et al., 2013). It is a diagnostic system that currently is used primarily for research settings but shows promise for use in clinical settings as well. The RDoC is a research framework developed by the National Institute of Mental Health (NIMH). It was first proposed in 2009 by Thomas Insel, the former director of NIMH (Cuthbert & Insel, 2013). When developing this system, Insel argued that the Diagnostic and Statistical Manual of Mental Disorders was outdated and not based on a sound understanding of the underlying biology or behavioral processes of these disorders. He proposed the RDoC as a new framework that would focus on those underlying processes that contribute to mental disorders.

For the first several years of the RDoC existence, it was used exclusively for research settings. In recent years there has been more consideration of this system for clinical settings as well. One of the main reasons for this, is reflected in the comprehensive text by McCarty (2020) and its subtitle "Insight from Animal Models". What McCarty presents is the argument that the RDoC offers more than other diagnostic systems because of its basis in comparative psychology research. Animal models present a conceptualization of psychological disorders based on behavioral, neurological, and genetic factors. These are all the main factors considered in comparative psychology research.

There are several advantages that the RDoC has over the DSM-5 (Stein & Reed, 2019) and ICD-11. First, it provides a more comprehensive and nuanced understanding of mental disorders by considering multiple dimensions of mental function and behavior. This allows for a more individualized and precise diagnosis that considers the unique mechanisms that underlie an individual's symptoms. Second, the RDoC framework provides a framework for understanding the neural and cognitive mechanisms that underlie mental disorders. This can lead to the development of more effective treatments that target these underlying mechanisms. Third, the RDoC framework encourages interdisciplinary collaboration between researchers in different fields, such as neuroscience, psychology, and psychiatry. This can lead to a more integrated and comprehensive understanding of mental disorders.

RDoC is a diagnostic method that is consistent with basic behavioral research and not just clinical research. It is consistent with the animal models that guide understanding of the causes of psychological conditions (Salamone & Correa, 2022) and not just the human models emphasized in clinical settings. When considered in this way, the RDoC presents a strong alternative to the DSM-5 because of its consistency with comparative psychology research and other areas of basic psychological research (Halpin, 2016). It is not only used in comparative psychology but is based on the research approach emphasized in comparative psychology. This system represents a very good example of the intersection of comparative psychology and clinical psychology. As such it also represents the best alternative for a diagnostic system consistent with the needs of this new field that we are calling comparative psychopathology.

Contribution Of Comparative Psychology to Understanding Psychopathology

Comparative psychopathology incorporates the contribution comparative psychology and the study of behavior across species offers for understanding psychological disorders. Its emphasis is on basic empirical research and what it shows about how psychological constructs function. The RDoC offers a diagnostic system that also emphasizes basic psychological research and what it shows about psychological constructs. To understand what benefit this system could have for clinical work it is useful to look briefly at some specific contributions comparative psychology research makes to understanding psychopathology.

One of the most important contributions of comparative psychology is the demonstration that psychological disorders are not unique to humans. This is something that has been understood in psychology since the work of I.P. Pavlov in the early 20th century (Pavlov, 2020). Many of the same symptoms and behaviors that we associate with psychological disorders can be seen in other animals. For example, anxiety (Ohl et al., 2008), depression (Lecorps et al., 2021), and aggressive disorders (Lischinsky & Lin, 2020) have all been observed in nonhuman animals. This suggests that the underlying causes of these disorders may be shared by humans and other animals.

Comparative psychology was also one of the first fields with research contributing to our understanding of the development of psychological disorders (Papini, 2020). Studies of animal models have shown how strongly early experiences can impact mental health. For example, understanding how exposure to stress or trauma in early life can increase the risk of developing anxiety or depression later in life (Agorastos et al., 2019). Studies of animal behaviors have been such a major part of the history of understanding psychopathology and its development that it is important to continue having it a major part of how it is currently understood.

Clinical research has become primary in understanding psychological treatments, but most professionals recognize its limitations. Research focusing on treating specific disorders with specific interventions is often too rigid, simplistic, and polished to have much value in real clinical settings. Interventions require not only an understanding of what works but also solid theory with research support about why they work (Haslbeck et al., 2022).

Having a diagnostic system that accounts not only for how disorders exist but also for why they exist would go a long way toward overcoming the limitations of present systems. Comparative psychology research on disorders focuses almost exclusively on the "why" rather than just the "what" when it comes to psychological disorders.

Finally, a diagnostic system that includes animal models as a way of understanding disorders would put clinical psychology more on par with medical treatments (Singh & Seed, 2021). Comparative psychology has contributed a great deal to animal models used in medicine. Medical treatments presently rely a great deal on animal models of disease and animal models are required to show how any medicines work. Most medicines cannot be approved unless their path of effectiveness shows consistency with animal models. Utilizing the RDoC would bring that same sort of requirement into the clinical psychology arena.

There is a real need for alternative diagnostic systems to the DSM-5. For too long the mental health profession has been satisfied with this system that provides almost no guidance for case conceptualization other than that connected to the pharmaceutical industry (Bandini, 2015; Cosgrove & Krimsky 2012; Cosgrove & Wheeler, 2013; Cosgrove et al., 2016; Roy et al., 2019; Sweet & Decoteau, 2018). Considering an approach to diagnoses, like the RDoC, which emphasizes psychology from the perspective of behavioral concepts along with neurology would bring back in line with the concepts emphasized since the founding of psychotherapy (Fernández-Álvarez et al., 2016).

How The RDoC Works

The RDoC is based on a dimensional approach to mental disorders, which considers the multiple dimensions of mental function and behavior. It was developed as a method that could use research in neurological and behavioral sciences to impact future diagnostic revisions more directly in systems like the DSM-5 (Cuthbert, 2022). However, even during its early stage of development, it was presented as a possible alternative to diagnostic systems already in use (Insel et al., 2010). Working with the method in terms of understanding psychopathology for research led to proposals that it be used as a diagnostic method itself.

This system is an approach to understanding mental illness that emphasizes the importance of studying underlying mechanisms of behavior across multiple levels of analysis, from molecular and cellular to neural circuits and behavior (Fernandez et al., 2016). These neural circuits could be caused by physiological factors or environmental ones. Genetics plays a major role in this conceptualization as does the impact of reward systems. Consideration of all these systems makes it consistent with comparative psychology as it allows for more focus on how these factors impact behavior and functioning across species (Nielsen et al., 2021).

RDoC is considered a "transdiagnostic" system and it is useful to look at this aspect of the RDoC before moving on to the practicalities of how it works. "Transdiagnostic" systems are ones that consider symptoms as they impact the development and maintenance of multiple disorders (Dalgleish et al., 2020). This is a different way of looking at disorders from systems like the DSM-5, where the emphasis is on the presence or absence of certain symptoms. Anxious and depressive disorders, for example, are described in the DSM-5 primarily only on the symptoms that distinguish the two types of disorders. This can cause difficulties since disorders like these often share similar symptoms. By looking at the degree to which different factors occur, rather than just whether these factors are present or not, transdiagnostic symptoms allow more room to look at ways the disorders might be both similar and different. By considering transdiagnostic systems in more detail a system like the RDoC allows for a more detailed focus on how anxiety and depressive disorder symptoms often overlap (Eysenck & Fajkowska, 2018; Gentes & Ruscio, 2011) and what steps allow for more detailed diagnoses.

There are six main domains in the RDoC framework. These domains are negative valence systems, positive valence systems, cognitive systems, social processes, arousal/regulatory systems, and sensorimotor systems. Research on the RDoC shows it is a very effective way of translating scientific behavioral and neuroscience research across species into a better understanding of human and nonhuman animal psychology. Five out of the six main domains have been found to fit both with understanding human and nonhuman animal psychological processes (Anderzhanova et al., 2017). "Cognitive systems" is the only domain to fit humans only as it includes a large language and abstract communication component. Each of the domains has several constructs that address different aspects of the domains and then some of those constructs have subconstructs.

Here is a list of the domains and constructs, along with definitions of each, taken from the RDoC Website (https://www.nimh.nih.gov/research/research-funded-by-nimh/rdoc/constructs/):

Domain: Negative Valence System
Definition: Primarily responsible for responses to aversive situations or contexts, such as fear, anxiety, and loss.
Acute Threat ("Fear")
Description: Activation of the brain's defensive motivational system to promote behaviors that protect the organism from perceived danger. Normal fear involves a pattern of adaptive responses to conditioned or unconditioned threat stimuli (exteroceptive or interoceptive). Fear can involve

internal representations and cognitive processing and can be modulated by a variety of factors.

Potential Threat ("Anxiety")

Description: Activation of a brain system in which harm may potentially occur but is distant, ambiguous, or low/uncertain in probability, characterized by a pattern of responses such as enhanced risk assessment (vigilance). These responses to low-imminence threats are qualitatively different than the high-imminence threat behaviors that characterize fear.

Sustained Threat

Description: An aversive emotional state caused by prolonged (i.e., weeks to months) exposure to internal and/or external condition(s), state(s), or stimuli that are adaptive to escape or avoid. The exposure may be actual or anticipated; the changes in affect, cognition, physiology, and behavior caused by sustained threat persist in the absence of the threat and can be differentiated from those changes evoked by acute threat.

Loss

Description: A state of deprivation of a motivationally significant conspecific, object, or situation. Loss may be social or non-social and may include permanent or sustained loss of shelter, behavioral control, status, loved ones, or relationships. The response to loss may be episodic (e.g., grief) or sustained.

Frustrative Non-Reward

Description: Reactions elicited in response to withdrawal/prevention of reward, i.e., by the inability to obtain positive rewards following repeated or sustained efforts.

Domain: Positive Valence Systems

Definition: Primarily responsible for responses to positive motivational situations or contexts, such as reward seeking, consummatory behavior, and reward/habit learning.

Reward Responsiveness

Description: Processes that govern an organism's hedonic response to impending or possible reward (as reflected in reward anticipation), the receipt of reward (as reflected in the initial response to reward), and following repeated receipt of reward (as in reward satiation); across these subdomains, reward responsiveness primarily reflects neural activity to receipt of reward and reward cues and can also be measured in terms of subjective and behavioral responses.

Reward Learning

Description: A process by which organisms acquire information about stimuli, actions, and contexts that predict positive outcomes, and by which behavior is modified when a novel reward occurs, or outcomes are better than expected. Reward learning is a type of reinforcement learning.

Reward Valuation

Description: Processes by which the probability and benefits of a prospective outcome are computed by reference to external information, social context (e.g., group input), and/or prior experience. This computation is influenced by preexisting biases, learning, memory, stimulus characteristics, and deprivation states. Reward valuation may involve the assignment of incentive salience to stimuli.

Domain: Cognitive Systems

Definition: Responsible for various cognitive processes.

Attention

Description: Attention refers to a range of processes that regulate access to capacity-limited systems, such as awareness, higher perceptual processes, and motor action. The concepts of capacity limitation and competition are inherent to the concepts of selective and divided attention.

Perception

Description: Perception refers to the process(es) that perform computations on sensory data to construct and transform representations of the external environment, acquire information from, and make predictions about, the external world, and guide action.

Declarative Memory

Description: Declarative memory is the acquisition or encoding, storage and consolidation, and retrieval of representations of facts and events. Declarative memory provides the critical substrate for relational representations—i.e., for spatial, temporal, and other contextual relations among items, contributing to representations of events (episodic memory) and the integration and organization of factual knowledge (semantic memory). These representations facilitate the inferential and flexible extraction of new information from these relationships.

Language

Description: Language is a system of shared symbolic representations of the world, the self, and abstract concepts that supports thought and communication.

Cognitive Control

Description: A system that modulates the operation of other cognitive and emotional systems, in the service of goal-directed behavior, when prepotent modes of responding are not adequate to meet the demands of the current context. Additionally, control processes are engaged in the case of novel contexts, where appropriate responses need to be selected from among competing alternatives.

Working Memory

Description: A system that modulates the operation of other cognitive and emotional systems, in the service of goal-directed behavior, when prepotent modes of responding are not adequate to meet the demands of the current context. Additionally, control processes are engaged in the case of novel contexts, where appropriate responses need to be selected from among competing alternatives.

Domain: Social Processes

Definition: Systems for Social Processes mediate responses in interpersonal settings of various types, including perception and interpretation of others' actions.

Affiliation and Attachment

Description: Affiliation is engagement in positive social interactions with other individuals. Attachment is selective affiliation as a consequence of the development of a social bond. Affiliation and Attachment are moderated by social information processing (processing of social cues) and social motivation. Affiliation is a behavioral consequence of social motivation and can manifest itself in social approach behaviors. Affiliation and Attachment require detection of and attention to social cues, as well as social learning and memory associated with forming relationships. Affiliation and Attachment include both the positive physiological consequences of social interactions and the behavioral and physiological consequences of disruptions to social relationships. Clinical manifestations of disruptions in Affiliation and Attachment include social withdrawal, social indifference and anhedonia, and over-attachment.

Social Communication

Definition: Social communication is a dynamic process that includes both receptive and productive aspects used to exchange socially relevant information. Social communication is essential for of integrating and maintaining the individual in the social environment. This construct is reciprocal and interactive, and social communication abilities may appear very early in life.

Social communication is distinguishable from other cognitive systems (e.g., perception, cognitive control, memory, attention) in that it particularly involves interactions with conspecifics. The underlying neural substrates of social communication evolved to support both automatic/reflexive and volitional control, including the motivation and ability to engage in social communication. Receptive aspects may be implicit or explicit; examples include affect recognition, facial recognition, and characterization. Productive aspects include eye contact, expressive reciprocation, and gaze following.

Perception and Understanding of Self

Definition: Perception and Understanding of Self includes the processes and/or representations involved in being aware of, accessing knowledge about, and/or making judgments about the self. These processes/

representations can include current cognitive or emotional internal states, traits, and/or abilities, either in isolation or in relationship to others, as well as the mechanisms that support self-awareness, self-monitoring, and self-knowledge.

Perception and Understanding of Others

Definition: Perception and Understanding of Others include the processes and/or representations involved in being aware of, accessing knowledge about, reasoning about, and/or making judgments about other animate entities, including information about cognitive or emotional states, traits, or abilities.

Domain: Arousal and Regulatory Systems

Definition: Arousal/Regulatory Systems are responsible for generating activation of neural systems as appropriate for various contexts and providing appropriate homeostatic regulation of such systems as energy balance and sleep.

Arousal

Definition: Arousal is a continuum of sensitivity of the organism to stimuli, both external and internal. Arousal facilitates interaction with the environment in a context-specific manner (e.g., under conditions of threat, some stimuli must be ignored while sensitivity to and responses to others is enhanced, as exemplified in the startle reflex). It can be evoked by either external/environmental stimuli or internal stimuli (e.g., emotions and cognition). It can be modulated by the physical characteristics and motivational significance of stimuli. It varies along a continuum that can be quantified in any behavioral state, including wakefulness and low-arousal states including sleep, anesthesia, and coma. Arousal is distinct from motivation and valence but can covary with intensity of motivation and valence. It may be associated with increased or decreased locomotor activity and can be regulated by homeostatic drives (e.g., hunger, sleep, thirst, sex).

Circadian Rhythms

Definition: Circadian rhythms are endogenous self-sustaining oscillations that organize the timing of biological systems to optimize physiology behavior, and health. They are synchronized by recurring environmental cues; anticipate the external environment; allow effective responses to challenges and opportunities in the physical and social environment; modulate homeostasis within the brain and other (central/peripheral) systems, tissues, and organs; are evident across levels of organization including molecules, cells, circuits, systems, organisms, and social systems.

Sleep-Wakefulness

Definition: Sleep and wakefulness are endogenous, recurring, behavioral states that reflect coordinated changes in the dynamic functional organization of the brain and that optimize physiology, behavior, and health.

Homeostatic and circadian processes regulate the propensity for wakefulness and sleep. Sleep is reversible, typically characterized by postural recumbence, behavioral quiescence, and reduced responsiveness. Sleep has a complex architecture with predictable cycling of NREM/REM states (or the developmental equivalent of NREM/REM states). NREM and REM sleep have distinct neural substrates (circuitry, transmitters, modulators) and EEG oscillatory properties. The intensity and duration of sleep are affected by homeostatic regulation and experiences during wakefulness. Sleep is evident at cellular, circuit, and system levels and has restorative and transformative effects that optimize neurobehavioral functions during wakefulness.

Domain: Sensorimotor Systems
Definition: Sensorimotor systems are primarily responsible for the control and execution of motor behaviors, and their refinement during learning and development.

Motor Actions
Definition: A multifaceted construct comprising the processes that must be engaged during the planning and execution of a motor action in a context-appropriate manner. Component processes include action planning and selection, sensorimotor dynamics, initiation, execution, and inhibition and termination. Of note, these processes will often be recruited in conjunction with motivational processes described in other domains, as when appetitive motivations drive approach behaviors. This construct explicitly includes the modulation and refinement of actions during development and learning. The list of subconstructs is not intended to imply a specific order or sequence.

Agency and Ownership
Definition: The sense that one is initiating, executing, and in control of one's volitional actions and their sensory consequences and the sense that one's body or body parts belong to oneself. This may include comparing the predicted and actual sensory consequences of one's action, awareness of the intention to move, temporal binding of self-generated action and their immediate effects, and attenuation of sensory consequences of self-generated actions.

Habit
Definition: Learned stimulus-response mappings triggered by internal or external stimuli that are autonomous of the current value of the outcome or goal. Habits may include overlearned sequences. Habits are implicit and efficient, requiring few cognitive resources, but can also be maladaptive under novel circumstances. Habits are based on previous positively or negatively reinforced learning and commonly occur after extended learning. Both habit formation and expression are commonly operationalized

within motor control systems. When habit formation is motivated by reward learning it overlaps with the Habit construct within the Positive Valence domain.

Using the RDOC for Clinical Settings

As can be seen from the above summary of domains and constructs, the RDoC presents a very useful for a very complex set of factors to consider when diagnosing. When using the system this diagnostic approach involves deciding which domains and constructs have the most importance for an individual case and then considering how that might match with factors important for certain diagnostic categories. Consideration of overlap between categories is also considered along with whether there may be an interaction of a diagnostic category being primary but other categories playing secondary roles. Typically the method used to illustrate this complexity is a sort of matrix although the formal system that might be used in a clinical setting is still being developed.

To address how this diagnostic system is used it would be helpful to look at examples of how it is applied for clinical conditions. Given their prominence in the clinical realm, depression, and schizophrenia are two clinical disorders worth looking at for considering how RDoC works.

When considering any diagnostic issue all domains are considered but one step is to try and identify what domains will likely be most important. In the case of depression, the negative valence systems domain is likely to be the most relevant (Dillon et al., 2014; Woody & Gibb, 2015) as it includes constructs related to negative emotions, such as sadness, anxiety, and fear. This approach would work both when considering a specific diagnosis (where the question would be what domains are most relevant) and specific clinical cases (where the question would be what domain seems to stand out in how the individual presents).

Once the main domains are identified, the next step is to assess the relevant constructs: Within the negative valence systems domain, several constructs are relevant to depression, including negative affect, loss, and potential threat. For example, a person with depression may experience persistent feelings of sadness and hopelessness (negative affect) and have a decreased interest in activities they previously enjoyed (loss).

After the main domains and constructs are identified the next step is to evaluate the severity and impact of symptoms: Using the RDoC framework, symptoms are evaluated on a continuum rather than being placed into discrete diagnostic categories. This means that the severity and impact of symptoms can be assessed more accurately. For example, a person with depression may have severe feelings of sadness and hopelessness that have a significant impact on their ability to function in daily life.

In this diagnostic process the last major step is to consider the role of underlying mechanisms: The RDoC framework emphasizes the importance of considering underlying mechanisms of functioning in mental disorders. For depression, this may include factors such as neurobiological changes in brain circuits involved in emotion regulation or stress response.

When considering schizophrenia, the steps for diagnosing with the RDoC are the same as depression. In the case of schizophrenia, the cognitive systems domain is likely to be the most relevant, as it includes constructs related to attention, working memory, cognitive control, and perception (Schwarz et al., 2016; Ford et al., 2014). Discussing perception would be important as this would be where unusual perceptual experiences evident in hallucinations or delusions would be identified.

Within the cognitive systems domain, several constructs are relevant to schizophrenia, including attention, working memory, cognitive flexibility, and perception. For example, a person with schizophrenia may experience deficits in attention, with difficulty focusing on relevant information and ignoring irrelevant stimuli.

Evaluating the severity of symptoms will depend on individual cases. For example, a person with schizophrenia may experience severe deficits in attention that significantly impact their ability to perform daily tasks and engage in social interactions. Notice that this measure of severity does not focus on whether the person has hallucinations or delusions but more on the impact that hallucinations or delusions have on the person being able to maintain attention.

Schizophrenia is considered primarily a neurological disorder, and this would mean that underlying neurological systems would be particularly important. For schizophrenia, this may include factors such as abnormalities in neural circuits involved in attention and perception, as well as changes in neurotransmitter systems such as dopamine and glutamate.

Using RDOC To Inform Animal Models

Applying the RDoc for clinical settings helps improve the use of animal models for understanding disorders. This helps improve the impact of animal models for addressing human psychopathology. If this was used more often in clinical settings it would allow the clinical use to improve the animal models. This would allow the RDoC to be more circular in terms of animal models being used for improving clinical work and then its use in clinical work to improve the quality of animal models.

Here are some ideas for how the RDoC can help inform animal models and make them more consistent with what is needed for clinical research:

- The RDoC framework can inform the development of animal models by identifying specific behavioral domains and constructs that are relevant to a given psychiatric disorder. For example, the RDoC framework includes a social processes domain that is relevant to disorders such as autism spectrum disorder and social anxiety disorder.

- Researchers using the RDoC can design animal models that more accurately reflect the underlying mechanisms of the disorder. For example, a mouse model of autism spectrum disorder may be designed to test deficits in social cognition or communication.
- Theoretical and research frameworks using the RDoC emphasize the importance of studying multiple levels of analysis, from molecular and cellular to neural circuits and behavior. Animal models can be used to investigate these levels of analysis in a more controlled manner than is possible in human studies. For example, animal models can be used to investigate the molecular and cellular mechanisms underlying changes in neural circuits and behavior that are associated with psychiatric disorders. This can lead to the identification of potential targets for new treatments.
- Research using the RDoC framework also emphasizes the importance of studying the interactions between different domains and constructs. Animal models can be used to investigate how changes in one domain or construct may impact other domains and constructs. For example, a mouse model of depression may be used to investigate how changes in negative valence systems, such as anhedonia or loss of motivation, may impact other domains, such as social processes or cognitive systems.
- Animal models can also be used to investigate the impact of environmental factors on the development and progression of psychiatric disorders. The RDoC framework emphasizes the importance of studying how environmental factors interact with genetic and biological factors to influence the development of mental illness. For example, animal models can be used to investigate how early life stress or exposure to environmental toxins may impact the development of neural circuits and behavior that are relevant to psychiatric disorders.
- The RDoC framework can inform the development of animal models by guiding the selection of outcome measures. The RDoC framework emphasizes the importance of using objective and quantitative measures of behavior and neural function. For example, animal models of anxiety disorders may be designed to test objective measures of fear or anxiety, such as changes in heart rate or freezing behavior.
- Animal models can also be used to investigate the efficacy and mechanisms of action of potential treatments for psychiatric disorders. The RDoC framework can guide the design of studies that test the effects of treatments on specific domains and constructs. For example, an animal model of schizophrenia may be used to test the effects of a potential new treatment on working memory deficits or alterations in dopamine signaling.

- The RDoC framework also emphasizes the importance of studying individual differences in the development and progression of psychiatric disorders. Animal models can be used to investigate how genetic and environmental factors interact to produce individual differences in behavior and neural function. For example, animal models can be used to investigate how genetic variations or epigenetic modifications may impact the development of neural circuits and behavior that are relevant to psychiatric disorders.

References

Agorastos, A., Pervanidou, P., Chrousos, G. P., & Baker, D. G. (2019). Developmental trajectories of early life stress and trauma: A narrative review on neurobiological aspects beyond stress system dysregulation. *Frontiers in Psychiatry, 10,* 118.

American Psychiatric Association. (2013). *Diagnostic and statistical manual of mental disorders* (5th ed.). Washington, DC: American Psychiatric Association.

Anderzhanova, E., Kirmeier, T., & Wotjak, C.T. (2017). Animal models in psychiatric research: The RDoC system as a new framework for endophenotype-oriented translational neuroscience. *Neurobiology of Stress, 7,* 47–56. https://doi.org/10.1016/j.ynstr.2017.03.003. PMID: 28377991; PMCID: PMC5377486.

Bandini, J. (2015). The medicalization of bereavement: (Ab)normal grief in the DSM-5. *Death Studies, 39*(6), 347–352.

Casey, B. J., Craddock, N., Cuthbert, B. N., Hyman, S. E., Lee, F. S., & Ressler, K. J. (2013). DSM-5 and RDoC: Progress in psychiatry research? *Nature Reviews Neuroscience, 14*(11), 810–814.

Cosgrove, L., & Krimsky, S. (2012). A comparison of DSM-IV and DSM-5 panel members' financial associations with industry: A pernicious problem persists. *PLoS Medicine, 9*(3), e1001190.

Cosgrove, L., & Wheeler, E. E. (2013). Industry's colonization of psychiatry: Ethical and practical implications of financial conflicts of interest in the DSM-5. *Feminism & Psychology, 23*(1), 93–106.

Cosgrove, V. E., Kelsoe, J. R., & Suppes, T. (2016). Toward a valid animal model of bipolar disorder: how the research domain criteria help bridge the clinical-basic science divide. *Biological psychiatry, 79*(1), 62–70.

Cuthbert, B. N. (2022). Research domain criteria (RDoC): Progress and potential. *Current Directions in Psychological Science, 31*(2), 107–114.

Cuthbert, B. N., & Insel, T. R. (2013). Toward the future of psychiatric diagnosis: The seven pillars of RDoC. *BMC Medicine, 11*(1), 1–8.

Dalgleish, T., Black, M., Johnston, D., & Bevan, A. (2020). Transdiagnostic approaches to mental health problems: Current status and future directions. *Journal of Consulting and Clinical Psychology, 88*(3), 179–195.

Dillon, D. G., Rosso, I. M., Pechtel, P., Killgore, W. D., Rauch, S. L., & Pizzagalli, D. A. (2014). Peril and pleasure: An RDOC-inspired examination of threat responses and reward processing in anxiety and depression. *Depression and Anxiety, 31*(3), 233–249.

Eysenck, M. W., & Fajkowska, M. (2018). Anxiety and depression: Toward overlapping and distinctive features. *Cognition and Emotion, 32*(7), 1391–1400.

Fernandez, K. C., Jazaieri, H., & Gross, J. J. (2016). Emotion regulation: A transdiagnostic perspective on a new RDoC domain. *Cognitive Therapy and Research, 40,* 426–440.

Fernández-Álvarez, H., Consoli, A. J., & Gómez, B. (2016). Integration in psychotherapy: Reasons and challenges. *American Psychologist*, *71*(8), 820.

First, M. B., Gaebel, W., Maj, M., Stein, D. J., Kogan, C. S., Saunders, J. B., & Reed, G. M. (2021). An organization-and category-level comparison of diagnostic requirements for mental disorders in ICD-11 and DSM-5. *World Psychiatry*, *20*(1), 34–51.

Ford, J. M., Morris, S. E., Hoffman, R. E., Sommer, I., Waters, F., McCarthy-Jones, S., & Cuthbert, B. N. (2014). Studying hallucinations within the NIMH RDoC framework. *Schizophrenia Bulletin*, *40*(Suppl_4), S295–S304.

Gaebel, W., Stricker, J., & Kerst, A. (2020). Changes from ICD-10 to ICD-11 and future directions in psychiatric classification. *Dialogues in Clinical Neuroscience*, *22*(1), 7–15. https://doi.org/10.31887/DCNS.2020.22.1/wgaebel. PMID: 32699501; PMCID: PMC7365296.

Gentes, E. L., Ruscio, A. M. (2011). A meta-analysis of the relation of intolerance of uncertainty to symptoms of generalized anxiety disorder, major depressive disorder, and obsessive–compulsive disorder. *Clinical Psychology Review*, *31*, 923–933. https://doi.org/10.1016/j.cpr.2011.05.001.

Halpin, M. (2016). The DSM and professional practice: Research, clinical, and institutional perspectives. *Journal of Health and Social Behavior*, *57*(2), 153–167.

Haslbeck, J., Ryan, O., Robinaugh, D. J., Waldorp, L. J., & Borsboom, D. (2022). Modeling psychopathology: From data models to formal theories. *Psychological Methods*, *27*(6), 930.

Hayes, S. C., Hofmann, S. G., & Ciarrochi, J. (2020). A process-based approach to psychological diagnosis and treatment: The conceptual and treatment utility of an extended evolutionary meta model. *Clinical Psychology Review*, *82*, 101908.

Insel, T., Cuthbert, B., Garvey, M., Heinssen, R., Pine, D. S., Quinn, K. & Wang, P. (2010). Research domain criteria (RDoC): Toward a new classification framework for research on mental disorders. *American Journal of Psychiatry*, *167*(7), 748–751.

Lasalvia, A. (2015). DSM-5 two years later: Facts, myths and some key open issues. *Epidemiology and Psychiatric Sciences*, *24*(3), 185–187.

Lecorps, B., Weary, D. M., & von Keyserlingk, M. A. (2021). Captivity-induced depression in animals. *Trends in Cognitive Sciences*, *25*(7), 539–541.

Lingiardi, V., McWilliams, N., Bornstein, R. F., Gazzillo, F., & Gordon, R. M. (2015). The Psychodynamic Diagnostic Manual Version 2 (PDM-2): Assessing patients for improved clinical practice and research. *Psychoanalytic Psychology*, *32*(1), 94.

Lischinsky, J. E., & Lin, D. (2020). Neural mechanisms of aggression across species. *Nature Neuroscience*, *23*(11), 1317–1328.

McCarty, R. (2020). *Stress and mental disorders: Insights from animal models*. London: Oxford Press.

Nielsen, A. N., Wakschlag, L. S., & Norton, E. S. (2021). Linking irritability and functional brain networks: A transdiagnostic case for expanding consideration of development and environment in RDoC. *Neuroscience & Biobehavioral Reviews*, *129*, 231–244.

Ohl, F., Arndt, S. S., & van der Staay, F. J. (2008). Pathological anxiety in animals. *The Veterinary Journal*, *175*(1), 18–26.

Papini, M. R. (2020). *Comparative psychology: Evolution and development of brain and behavior*. New York: Routledge.

Pavlov, I. P. (2020). Experimental psychology and psychopathology in animals. In: *Psychopathology and psychiatry* (pp. 13–30). New York: Routledge.

PDM Task Force. (2006). *Psychodynamic diagnostic manual*. Silver Spring, MD: Alliance of Psychoanalytic Organizations.

Roy, M., Rivest, M. P., Namian, D., & Moreau, N. (2019). The critical reception of the DSM-5: Towards a typology of audiences. *Public Understanding of Science*, *28*(8), 932–948.

Salamone, J. D., & Correa, M. (2022). Critical review of RDoC approaches to the study of motivation with animal models: Effort valuation/willingness to work. *Emerging Topics in Life Sciences*, *6*(5), 515–528.

Schwarz, E., Tost, H., & Meyer-Lindenberg, A. (2016). Working memory genetics in schizophrenia and related disorders: An RDoC perspective. *American Journal of Medical Genetics Part B: Neuropsychiatric Genetics*, *171*(1), 121–131.

Shorter, E. (2022). The history of nosology and the rise of the Diagnostic and Statistical Manual of Mental Disorders. *Dialogues in Clinical Neuroscience*.

Singh, V. K., & Seed, T. M. (2021). How necessary are animal models for modern drug discovery? *Expert Opinion on Drug Discovery*, *16*(12), 1391–1397.

Stein, D. J., & Reed, G. M. (2019). Global mental health and psychiatric nosology: DSM-5, ICD-11, and RDoC. *Brazilian Journal of Psychiatry*, *41*, 3–4.

Sweet, P. L., & Decoteau, C. L. (2018). Contesting normal: The DSM-5 and psychiatric subjectivation. *BioSocieties*, *13*, 103–122.

Woody, M. L., & Gibb, B. E. (2015). Integrating NIMH research domain criteria (RDoC) into depression research. *Current Opinion in Psychology*, *4*, 6–12.

3 Social Competition Theory and Clinical Depression

Introduction

According to the World Health Organization (WHO), depression is the leading cause of disability worldwide. It is also estimated that depression ranks second in Years Lived with a Disability (World Health Organization, 2021). Clinical depression is the most common mental disorder in the world, affecting over 264 million people across the globe. In the United States, about 16.2 million adults (or 6.7%) experienced at least one major depressive episode in 2020. Costs for depression treatment and its economic impact on impacted households increase dramatically in economic problems for people living in impoverished countries (Hailemichael et al., 2019).

Because of its prevalence, depression needs to be a major focus of any diagnostic system. Being able to identify the symptoms of depression, where they fit in terms of major psychological constructs and ways that the symptoms cluster together for different diagnoses are essential purposes of diagnostic systems. Considering comparative psychopathology as a valid system for understanding mental health disorders requires a means of explaining depressive symptomology and depressive disorders.

What we will see in this system is that comparative psychopathology as a diagnostic approach addresses one of the major limitations associated with diagnostic symptoms, the lack of emphasis on cause (Kountouras & Sotirgiannidou, 2022). Comparative psychopathology looks to incorporate psychological research into an understanding of what factors need to be considered when defining diagnostic categories. As will be shown in this chapter on depression, again one of the most common psychological disorders, the emphasis is not on changing what words are used to identify diagnoses. What is changed is an emphasis on defining these words not just in terms of the symptoms associated with them but also in an understanding of why those symptoms exist.

DOI: 10.4324/9781003408918-4

Several main theories attempt to explain the complex nature of clinical depression. The biological theories propose that imbalances in neurotransmitters, particularly serotonin, norepinephrine, and dopamine, play a significant role in the development of depression (Kennis et al., 2020; Moncrieff et al., 2022). This theory is supported by evidence of the effectiveness of antidepressant medications that target these neurotransmitters. The cognitive theories posit that negative thinking patterns and distorted cognitive processes contribute to depression (Mohammadkhani et al., 2020). It suggests that individuals with depression tend to interpret events and experiences in a negative and self-deprecating manner, leading to a cycle of negative emotions and behaviors. The psychodynamic theories focus on unresolved conflicts and unconscious processes, suggesting that depression can arise from repressed feelings, unresolved childhood issues, or internalized anger or guilt (Ribeiro et al., 2017). The sociocultural theories emphasize the impact of social and cultural factors on depression, such as stressful life events, social isolation, societal expectations, and cultural norms. It highlights the influence of social support, socioeconomic status, and cultural beliefs in the development and manifestation of depression (Hyde & Mezulis, 2020).

Introduction To Social Competition Theory

For a comparative psychopathology approach to understanding depression, the sociocultural theories offer the most direct explanations, One of the most prominent theories in the category of sociocultural theories is social competition theory. This theory arises straight from comparative psychology research (Price et al., 1994). This theory offers a perspective on how social dynamics and competitive interactions contribute to the development of clinical depression. Social competition theory was first proposed by Price (1967) and has been further developed by others, such as Fournier et al. (2007). According to this theory, depression evolved as an adaptive strategy to help individuals avoid social conflict and maintain their social status.

According to social competition theory, individuals are engaged in constant social comparisons and competition for resources, status, and social acceptance. In situations where individuals consistently experience social defeat, rejection, or perceive themselves as socially inferior, it can undermine their self-esteem, sense of belonging, and overall well-being (Wilson et al., 2020). This chronic exposure to social competition and feelings of inadequacy can activate the body's stress response, leading to dysregulation of stress hormones and neurotransmitters associated with depression. Moreover, negative cognitive biases associated with social competition, such as self-critical thoughts, excessive rumination, and perceived social threats, can further contribute to the development and maintenance of depressive symptoms. Overall, social competition theory suggests that the experience of social defeat, the pressure of social comparisons, and the resulting negative cognitive and emotional responses can significantly impact an individual's vulnerability to clinical depression.

Social competition theory is a framework that seeks to explain various aspects of human behavior by examining the influence of competition within social groups. According to this theory, individuals engage in competitive behaviors to gain and maintain social status, resources, and reproductive opportunities (Abele et al., 2021). It suggests that competition is an innate and pervasive aspect of human social interactions and plays a crucial role in shaping our thoughts, emotions, and actions. When seen this way social competition presents an avenue for understanding the development of and maintenance of depressive symptoms.

Social competition theory shows that individuals, both human and nonhuman, function In ways that try to show that they are outperforming other members of their social group. At its core, this theory posits that individuals are driven by the desire to outperform their peers and attain higher status within their social group (Walton et al., 2020). In human beings, this can manifest in various forms, such as academic achievements, career success, physical attractiveness, or material possessions. The theory argues that competition arises from the limited availability of resources, which creates a hierarchical structure where individuals strive to climb the social ladder and secure advantageous positions. What individuals seek to do is find a way that allows them to perceive that they are in a better place to get what they need from these limited resources.

This theory emphasizes the role of both intrasexual and intersexual competition. Intrasexual competition refers to competition between members of the same sex, typically for access to mates or resources. This can involve direct physical or verbal confrontations, as well as more subtle forms of competition, such as displays of prowess or dominance. Intersexual competition, on the other hand, involves competition between members of opposite sexes, usually in the context of attracting mates. It often takes the form of displaying desirable traits, engaging in conspicuous consumption, or engaging in acts of altruism to signal one's fitness as a potential partner.

Given that individuals, according to this theory, are trying to find ways of being at a higher rank than others it is important how that rank is communicated. One key aspect of social competition theory is the notion of signaling (Witkower et al., 2020). Individuals engage in competitive behaviors as a way to signal their qualities and capabilities to others. By excelling in a particular domain, they not only enhance their own social status but also communicate their fitness and suitability as potential mates, allies, or rivals (Kromidha & Li, 2019). This signaling process is crucial for establishing and maintaining social hierarchies, as it allows individuals to evaluate and compare themselves to others within the group. Signaling plays a major role in clinical depression because it is the way that social rank is communicated to an individual.

Notice here how signaling connects with the idea of irrational thinking as a factor in depression. Cognitive theories of depression stress the role of irrational thinking in developing and maintaining clinical depression (Chan & Sun, 2021). Note that signaling reflects ways that social hierarchy is communicated but it is not the case that the communication has to be factually correct (Peckre et al., 2019). Individuals can interpret in irrational ways what is being signaled about where they stand compared to others and this can lead to the sort of irrational thinking about how one compares to others, and the importance of how they compare, which is often a problem in clinical depression.

It is also important to consider here that irrational thinking would be a reflection of signaling for humans, but it is not the only means of signaling. Nonhuman animals have a variety of means for signaling that, of course, do not involve words or other means of communication. This is a construct that crosses over between species and shows how important it is for all animals, human and nonhuman alike, to try and make themselves look favorably to others. When that does not happen it can cause a major blow to how a person sees themselves and leads to a sense of failure that is commonly associated with clinical depression.

Social Defeat and Clinical Depression

Social competition emphasizes the desire of individuals to obtain higher ranking within their social groups. In this theory, it is expected that when things are working out how the individual wants that individual signals sufficiently to obtain a desirable social status. Problems occur for the individual when that does not occur. When signaling shows that the individual is unable or unlikely to obtain the status they desire it often causes a strong sense of defeat. In social competition theory as applied to humans, clinical depression is thought to be triggered by experiences of social defeat, such as losing a job, being rejected by a romantic partner, or being bullied. These experiences can lead to a loss of social status, which can activate the depressive response. Social defeat is seen as being at the heart of what leads to social competition causing depression.

Social defeat, referring to experiences of being consistently overpowered or dominated by others in social interactions, can significantly contribute to the development of depression (Björkqvist, 2001). Depression impacted by experiences of social defeat has been shown throughout human and nonhuman animals, particularly rodent, studies (Carnevali et al., 2020; Heshmati et al., 2020). When individuals repeatedly face situations where they feel socially inferior, powerless, or rejected, it can erode their self-esteem, sense of belonging, and overall well-being.

There is a considerable body of research showing that social defeat plays a role in the development of clinical depression (Fakhoury et al., 2022). For example, studies have found that people with depression are more likely to have experienced social defeat in their lives (Hollis & Kabbaj, 2014). Additionally, research has shown that exposing animals to social defeat can lead to depressive-like symptoms (Yoshida et al., 2021). This research area shows the crossover between constructs important for the healthy functioning of both human and nonhuman animals. When there is a sense of social defeat and not obtaining a desired level of social positioning is signaled the individual shows signs of hopelessness and giving up, including lack of behavioral effort, social withdrawal, and poor eating (Toyoda, 2017).

Social defeat leads to behaviors consistent with clinical depression not just in terms of how the individual interprets their status but also on how others respond to their status. Signaling not only impacts how an individual interprets their situation but also how others interpret their social standing. As a result, social defeat leads to depression through the disruption of social relationships. When an individual is defeated in a social interaction, they may be more likely to withdraw from social interactions in the future. This social withdrawal can lead to loneliness, isolation, and a sense of social isolation, which can all contribute to the development of depression.

Social defeat impacts not only directly how others act toward individuals but also how the individual expects others to act toward them. Social defeat is considered a major factor in the depressive symptoms exhibited often by humans who suffer strokes (Lowry & Jin, 2020). Studies have shown that social defeat impacts not only how the individual responds to stressors in their immediate environment but also how they respond to future stressors (de Jong et al., 2005). It is this impact on perception and not just on reality that helps social defeat explain the longstanding impact of depression.

Research on rodents shows that even one episode of social defeat can lead an individual to withdraw and act defeated for an extended time period (Isovich et al., 2001). Repetitive social defeat has even more of an impact (Ver Hoeve et al., 2013). Multiple episodes of social defeat have a lasting effect shown not only in defeatist behaviors but also in neurological changes (Fanous et al., 2010; Hollis et al., 2010). This impact is seen not only in continuous social defeats but also in intermittent periods of social defeat. Considering the social defeat is important when studying clinical depression because of its lasting impact. What separates clinical depression apart from basic sadness is not just the extent of symptoms but also that the symptoms do not go away when the sad situation ends. Explaining clinical depression as a construct requires being able to show why the symptoms do not end when situations contributing to the emotional distress subside.

Biology and Social Competition

Research supporting the social competition theory of depression shows not only how social defeat contributes to behavioral outcomes consistent with depression but also factors that keep it impact in place. Social defeat leads to behaviors arising to reflect that the individual has learned where it expects to stand in the social hierarchy. This has a survival benefit as it would help the individual avoid fights with opponents who could seriously harm, or even kill, the individual. To maintain survival, the individual must show their defeatist stance to avoid other battles. It is even possible that the defeatist stance will help the individual avoid any battles and allow them to maintain survival by giving up before the battles even start. This survival benefit to taking a defeatist stance can be one reason why social defeat has such a lasting effect and why depressive symptoms associated with social defeat last longer than the presence of problem situations would suggest.

Social competition in general is also associated with biological factors explaining what would keep its impact in place. One important aspect is the role of hormones, particularly testosterone. Testosterone is known to play a significant role in modulating competitive behaviors, as it is associated with traits such as aggression, dominance, and the drive to seek social status (Castro & Edwards, 2016). It is seen as the neurochemical most associated with keeping social competition and social rank-seeking in place. Research findings support that testosterone functions as a competition hormone that calibrates psychological systems to current social standing and adaptively guides status-seeking efforts (Cheng & Kornienko, 2020). Studies have found that testosterone levels tend to increase in response to competitive situations, promoting assertiveness and competitive motivation. However, the relationship between testosterone and competition is complex and can vary depending on contextual factors and individual differences (Gleason et al., 2009).

Neurotransmitters also play a crucial role in the biology of social competition. This has shown the complexity of neurology and its impact on depression. Dopamine, a neurotransmitter strongly associated with depression, is a good example. It is typically described as being a neurochemical associated directly with clinical depression, but what its real impact is on reward and motivation. As such, it has been implicated in the experience of winning and the pursuit of social rewards. This would include pursuing social rewards associated with the individual perceiving they have reached a higher social rank (Wetherall et al., 2019). Winning a competition can release dopamine in the brain's reward system, reinforcing competitive behaviors and motivating individuals to continue seeking social success.

Serotonin, another neurotransmitter strongly associated with clinical depression, has been linked to social hierarchies and the regulation of social behaviors. Like dopamine, it is not directly related to clinical depression but is linked strongly to an individual's ability to calculate their social rank (Janet et al., 2022). Regulation of social hierarchy learning by serotonin transporter availability. Imbalances in serotonin levels have been associated with changes in aggression, social dominance, and subordination.

Research on these neurotransmitters, dopamine and serotonin, provides direct evidence of how the social competition theory deserves a dominant place in understanding clinical depression. They help show not only where the behaviors associated with depression come from but, more importantly, what keeps them in place. Given that dopamine and serotonin have for decades been strongly associated with clinical depression, this theory fits in with what has already been understood about clinical depression. Still, it adds even more than what previous theories provide. Again this would be evidence beyond explaining where the symptoms come from but why they do not go away when a depressive situation seems to end. Dopamine is what provides the reward mechanism for why determining social rank is so important. Serotonin provides how the individual calculates their social rank. Having a means by which the individual calculates social rank is important for survival as it helps the individual avoid injury by getting into conflicts with other individuals who are likely to harm or kill them (Schafer & Schiller, 2022).

Furthermore, brain regions involved in social cognition and emotion regulation are also implicated in the biology of social competition. The prefrontal cortex, amygdala, and insula are among the brain regions that are activated during competitive interactions (Colyn et al., 2019; DiMenichi & Tricomi, 2017; Tanuma et al., 2022). These areas are involved in processing social information, assessing social hierarchies, evaluating rewards and punishments, and regulating emotional responses. Dysfunction in these brain regions can contribute to altered social behaviors and responses to competition. It is very relevant here that each of these brain areas are ones considered associated with clinical depression.

Genetic factors also play a role in the biology of social competition (Clutton-Brock, 2021). Studies have identified genetic variations that are associated with individual differences in competitive tendencies, such as the COMT gene (Filipenko et al., 2002) and the MAOA gene (Newman et al., 2005). These genes are involved in the regulation of neurotransmitters and have been linked to traits such as aggression and risk-taking, which can influence competitive behaviors. Genetic research also shows that certain gene expressions can both make individuals more susceptible to the impact of single episodes of social defeat and also chronic social defeat (Reshetnikov et al., 2021).

Overall, the biology of social competition involves a complex interplay between hormones, neurotransmitters, brain regions, and genetic factors. These biological mechanisms influence our motivation, behavior, and emotional responses during competitive interactions, shaping the dynamics of social competition in humans and other animals. Social defeat activates the body's stress response, triggering the release of stress hormones, which, over time, can dysregulate the brain's reward and pleasure pathways. These neurobiological changes can lead to a decrease in the production of mood-regulating neurotransmitters like serotonin, contributing to depressive symptoms. Furthermore, social defeat can lead to negative cognitive biases, where individuals interpret social interactions and situations in a pessimistic and self-deprecating manner, reinforcing feelings of worthlessness and hopelessness. The social isolation and withdrawal often associated with depression can further perpetuate the cycle of social defeat, creating a vicious cycle that exacerbates depressive symptoms.

Conclusion

Notice here that the social competition theory, considered primarily a sociological theory of depression, actually spans all the theories of depression. This chapter addressed the neurological factors associated with clinical depression that are considered parts of the neurological theories of depression. Social competition and particularly social defeat signals lower social status and leads to behaviors consistent with depression. In humans, these behavioral responses are reflected in the self-statements and other types of negative cognitive responses associated with the cognitive theories of depression. Even the affective responses related to social defeat and the strive for social dominance led to the emotional responses typically associated with the psychodynamic theories of depression. Here it is particularly useful to consider that the founder of the psychodynamic movement in psychotherapy, Sigmund Freud, emphasized a great deal of the work of comparative psychologists of his day (Perkins-McVey, 2022).

Social competition theory serves as a bridge between comparative psychology and clinical psychology by providing a framework to understand the interplay between social dynamics, competition, and psychological well-being across species. In comparative psychology, the theory helps researchers explore how competition influences behavior, social hierarchies, mating strategies, and cooperation in different species. By studying the adaptive value of competitive behaviors, comparative psychologists gain insights into the evolutionary origins and functions of these behaviors. In clinical psychology, social competition theory sheds light on how the experience of competition, social comparison, and social defeat can contribute to the development of psychological disorders, including depression, anxiety, and low self-esteem. It highlights the impact of social factors on mental health and helps clinicians understand the role of competition-related stress, social isolation, and negative cognitive biases in psychological distress. By integrating principles from comparative psychology with clinical psychology, social competition theory offers a comprehensive understanding of how social dynamics and competition influence mental health and well-being in both humans and other animals.

References

Abele, A. E., Ellemers, N., Fiske, S. T., Koch, A., & Yzerbyt, V. (2021). Navigating the social world: Toward an integrated framework for evaluating self, individuals, and groups. *Psychological Review*, *128*(2), 290–314.

Björkqvist, K. (2001). Social defeat is a stressor in humans. *Physiology & Behavior*, *73*(3), 435–442.

Carnevali, L., Montano, N., Tobaldini, E., Thayer, J. F., & Sgoifo, A. (2020). The contagion of social defeat stress: Insights from rodent studies. *Neuroscience & Biobehavioral Reviews*, *111*, 12–18.

Castro, K. V., & Edwards, D. A. (2016). Testosterone, cortisol, and human competition. *Hormones and Behavior*, *82*, 21–37.

Chan, H. W. Q., & Sun, C. F. R. (2021). Irrational beliefs, depression, anxiety, and stress among university students in Hong Kong. *Journal of American College Health*, *69*(8), 827–841.

Cheng, J. T., & Kornienko, O. (2020). The neurobiology of human social behavior: A review of how testosterone and cortisol underpin competition and affiliation dynamics. *Salivary Bioscience: Foundations of Interdisciplinary Saliva Research and Applications*, 519–553.

Clutton-Brock, T. (2021). Social evolution in mammals. *Science*, *373*(6561), eabc9699.

Colyn, L., Venzala, E., Marco, S., Perez-Otaño, I., & Tordera, R. M. (2019). Chronic social defeat stress induces sustained synaptic structural changes in the prefrontal cortex and amygdala. *Behavioural brain research*, *373*, 112079.

de Jong, J. G., van der Vegt, B. J., Buwalda, B., & Koolhaas, J. M. (2005). Social environment determines the long-term effects of social defeat. *Physiology & Behavior*, *84*(1), 87–95.

DiMenichi, B. C., & Tricomi, E. (2017). Increases in brain activity during social competition predict decreases in working memory performance and later recall. *Human Brain Mapping*, *38*(1), 457–471.

Fakhoury, M., Fritz, M., & Sleiman, S. F. (2022). Behavioral paradigms for assessing cognitive functions in the chronic social Defeat stress model of depression. In: *Translational Research Methods for Major Depressive Disorder* (pp. 147–164). New York, NY: Springer US.

Fanous, S., Hammer Jr, R. P., & Nikulina, E. M. (2010). Short-and long-term effects of intermittent social defeat stress on brain-derived neurotrophic factor expression in mesocorticolimbic brain regions. *Neuroscience*, *167*(3), 598–607.

Filipenko, M. L., Beylina, A. G., Alekseyenko, O. V., Timofeeva, O. A., Avgustinovich, D. F., & Kudryavtseva, N. N. (2002). Association between the brain COMT gene expression and aggressive experience in daily agonistic confrontations in male mice. *Stress: Neural, Endocrine and Molecular Studies*, 157–161.

Fournier, M. A., Zuroff, D. C., & Moskowitz, D. S. (2007). The social competition theory of depression: Gaining from an evolutionary approach to losing. *Journal of Social and Clinical Psychology*, *26*(7), 786–790. https://doi.org/10.1521/jscp.2007.26.7.786

Gleason, E. D., Fuxjager, M. J., Oyegbile, T. O., & Marler, C. A. (2009). Testosterone release and social context: When it occurs and why. *Frontiers in Neuroendocrinology*, *30*(4), 460–469.

Hailemichael, Y., Hanlon, C., Tirfessa, K., Docrat, S., Alem, A., Medhin, G. & Hailemariam, D. (2019). Catastrophic health expenditure and impoverishment in households of persons with depression: A cross-sectional, comparative study in rural Ethiopia. *BMC Public Health*, *19*(1), 1–13.

Heshmati, M., Christoffel, D. J., LeClair, K., Cathomas, F., Golden, S. A., Aleyasin, H & Russo, S. J. (2020). Depression and social defeat stress are associated with inhibitory synaptic changes in the nucleus accumbens. *Journal of Neuroscience*, *40*(32), 6228–6233.

Hollis, F., & Kabbaj, M. (2014). Social defeat as an animal model for depression. *ILAR Journal*, *55*(2), 221–232.

Hollis, F., Wang, H., Dietz, D., Gunjan, A., & Kabbaj, M. (2010). The effects of repeated social defeat on long-term depressive-like behavior and short-term histone modifications in the hippocampus in male Sprague–Dawley rats. *Psychopharmacology*, *211*, 69–77.

Hyde, J. S., & Mezulis, A. H. (2020). Gender differences in depression: Biological, affective, cognitive, and sociocultural factors. *Harvard Review of Psychiatry*, *28*(1), 4–13.

Isovich, E., Engelmann, M., Landgraf, R., & Fuchs, E. (2001). Social isolation after a single defeat reduces striatal dopamine transporter binding in rats. *European Journal of Neuroscience*, *13*(6), 1254–1256.

Janet, R., Ligneul, R., Losecaat-Vermeer, A. B., Philippe, R., Bellucci, G., Derrington, E. & Dreher, J. C. (2022). Regulation of social hierarchy learning by serotonin transporter availability. *Neuropsychopharmacology*, *47*(13), 2205–2212.

Kennis, M., Gerritsen, L., van Dalen, M., Williams, A., Cuijpers, P., & Bockting, C. (2020). Prospective biomarkers of major depressive disorder: A systematic review and meta-analysis. *Molecular Psychiatry*, *25*(2), 321–338.

Kountouras, G., & Sotirgiannidou, K. (2022). Psychodiagnostic classification systems: A critical view. *International Journal of Social Science Research and Review*, *5*(4), 30–40.

Kromidha, E., & Li, M. C. (2019). Determinants of leadership in online social trading: A signaling theory perspective. *Journal of Business Research*, *97*, 184–197.

Lowry, C. A., & Jin, A. Y. (2020). Improving the social relevance of experimental stroke models: Social isolation, social defeat stress and stroke outcome in animals and humans. *Frontiers in Neurology*, *11*, 427.

Mohammadkhani, P., Bagheri, M., Dobson, K. S., Eskandari, E., Dejman, M., Bass, J., & Abdi, F. (2020). Negative thoughts in depression: A study in Iran. *International Journal of Psychology*, *55*(1), 83–89.

Moncrieff, J., Cooper, R. E., Stockmann, T., Amendola, S., Hengartner, M. P., & Horowitz, M. A. (2022). The serotonin theory of depression: A systematic umbrella review of the evidence. *Molecular Psychiatry*, 1–14.

Newman, T. K., Syagailo, Y. V., Barr, C. S., Wendland, J. R., Champoux, M., Graessle, M., ... & Lesch, K. P. (2005). Monoamine oxidase A gene promoter variation and rearing experience influences aggressive behavior in rhesus monkeys. *Biological Psychiatry*, *57*(2), 167–172.

Peckre, L., Kappeler, P. M., & Fichtel, C. (2019). Clarifying and expanding the social complexity hypothesis for communicative complexity. *Behavioral Ecology and Sociobiology*, *73*, 1–19.

Perkins-McVey, M. (2022). A portrait of the neurophysiologist as a young man: Claus, Darwin, and Sigmund Freud's search for the testes of the eel (1875–1877). *History of Psychology*.

Price, J., Sloman, L., Gardner, R., Gilbert, P., & Rohde, P. (1994). The social competition hypothesis of depression. *The British Journal of Psychiatry*, *164*(3), 309–315.

Price, J. S. (1967). Hypothesis: The dominance hierarchy and the evolution of mental illness. *Lancet*, ii, 243–246.

Reshetnikov, V. V., Kisaretova, P. E., Ershov, N. I., Merkulova, T. I., & Bondar, N. P. (2021). Social defeat stress in adult mice causes alterations in gene expression, alternative splicing, and the epigenetic landscape of H3K4me3 in the prefrontal cortex: An impact of early-life stress. *Progress in Neuro-Psychopharmacology and Biological Psychiatry*, *106*, 110068.

Ribeiro, Â., Ribeiro, J. P., & von Doellinger, O. (2017). Depression and psychodynamic psychotherapy. *Brazilian Journal of Psychiatry*, *40*, 105–109.

Schafer, M., & Schiller, D. (2022). A dominant role for serotonin in the formation of human social hierarchies. *Neuropsychopharmacology*, *47*(13), 2177–2178.

Tanuma, M., Niu, M., Ohkubo, J., Ueno, H., Nakai, Y., Yokoyama, Y. & Kasai, A. (2022). Acute social defeat stress activated neurons project to the claustrum and basolateral amygdala. *Molecular Brain*, *15*(1), 1–11.

Toyoda, A. (2017). Social defeat models in animal science: What we have learned from rodent models. *Animal Science Journal*, *88*(7), 944–952.

Ver Hoeve, E. S., Kelly, G., Luz, S., Ghanshani, S., & Bhatnagar, S. (2013). Short-term and long-term effects of repeated social defeat during adolescence or adulthood in female rats. *Neuroscience*, *249*, 63–73.

Walton, C. C., Baranoff, J., Gilbert, P., & Kirby, J. (2020). Self-compassion, social rank, and psychological distress in athletes of varying competitive levels. *Psychology of Sport and Exercise*, *50*, 101733.

Wetherall, K., Robb, K. A., & O'Connor, R. C. (2019). Social rank theory of depression: A systematic review of self-perceptions of social rank and their relationship with depressive symptoms and suicide risk. *Journal of Affective Disorders*, *246*, 300–319.

Wilson, M. W., Ridlon, A. D., Gaynor, K. M., Gaines, S. D., Stier, A. C., & Halpern, B. S. (2020). Ecological impacts of human-induced animal behaviour change. *Ecology Letters*, *23*(10), 1522–1536.

Witkower, Z., Tracy, J. L., Cheng, J. T., & Henrich, J. (2020). Two signals of social rank: Prestige and dominance are associated with distinct nonverbal displays. *Journal of Personality and Social Psychology*, *118*(1), 89.

World Health Organization. (2021). *Brief model disability survey: 2019 results for India*. Lao People's Democratic Republic and Tajikistan.

Yoshida, K., Drew, M. R., Kono, A., Mimura, M., Takata, N., & Tanaka, K. F. (2021). Chronic social defeat stress impairs goal-directed behavior through dysregulation of ventral hippocampal activity in male mice. *Neuropsychopharmacology*, *46*(9), 1606–1616.

4 Beyond the Basics of Anxiety Disorder

A Comparative Psychopathology Perspective

Introduction

Anxiety disorders stand out as prevalent and most common among psychiatric conditions, with a yearly impact on 18% of the population (Kessler et al., 2005; Stein et al., 2017). Their pervasive nature extends across various psychiatric disorders, often emerging in childhood and persisting throughout one's lifetime, causing enduring distress and impairment. Data from the National Comorbidity Survey Replication study underscores a notable 12-month prevalence of 18%, with a distinct two-to-one female prevalence in the reproductive years. Even in children and adolescents, the estimated lifetime prevalence of anxiety disorders ranges between 15% and 20% (Bateson et al., 2011).

Despite the availability of effective pharmacological and psychotherapeutic interventions, a considerable number of individuals fail to achieve substantial improvement. Recognizing the clinical significance of anxiety across diverse psychiatric conditions serves as a predictive factor for unfavorable outcomes. Addressing this challenge calls for a deeper exploration of the underlying brain mechanisms, providing a foundation for the development of neuroscientifically informed treatment approaches aimed at improving the long-term well-being of individuals grappling with significant anxiety.

The DSM-5 classification of anxiety now includes separation anxiety disorder, selective mutism, social anxiety disorder, panic disorder, agoraphobia, Generalized Anxiety Disorder (GAD), substance/medication-induced anxiety disorder, and anxiety disorder due to another medical condition (American Psychiatric Association, 2013).

Comparative Approach to Understanding Anxiety Disorders

The comparative approach involves the examination of different species or populations within a species to understand the ecological factors influencing behavior and to test hypotheses about function. Psychiatrists commonly

DOI: 10.4324/9781003408918-5

utilize evidence from other species, particularly in the study of anxiety mechanisms. Anxiety-Related Responses (ALR) observed in various animal species comprise increased heart rate, stress hormone release, restlessness, vigilance, fear of perilous environments, reduced feeding, exploratory behavior, and an increased inclination to interpret ambiguous stimuli as threatening (Brilot et al., 2010; Burman et al., 2009).

In Belding's study (Mateo, 2007) of ground squirrels, it was found that populations confronting higher predation levels exhibit more pronounced elements of the ALR. Variations in stress hormones between high- and low-predation environments become apparent shortly after the emergence of pups from the nest. This indicates that the ALR serves the function of detecting and managing threats, specifically from predators. The physiological, cognitive, and behavioral changes linked to the ALR are interpreted as adaptive responses fulfilling this function.

Cognitive alterations enhance the early detection of impending threats, and on a physiological level, the ALR readies the body for action by improving oxygenation, directing blood to muscles, and inducing sweating to cool the skin. Therefore, both the contexts in which anxious symptoms manifest and the nature of these symptoms support the view that anxiety functions to prepare, in physiological, cognitive, and behavioral terms, for the detection and management of threats to survival (Bateson et al., 2011). A paradigm has been seen where human anxiety aligns with the ALR observed in diverse species, sharing a common purpose of threat detection and preparation. This conceptual framework suggests a shared evolutionary purpose of threat detection and preparation, prompting.

Translational Relevant of Literature Review Findings from Animal Models to Human Anxiety Disorders

The translational relevance of research findings from animal models to human anxiety disorders is a pivotal aspect of advancing our understanding of the condition. Animal studies have provided crucial insights that have not only deepened our comprehension of anxiety mechanisms but have also paved the way for developing more effective interventions for humans (Griebel et al., 2002; Santarelli et al., 2003).

Several studies highlight the successful translation of knowledge gained from animal models to human anxiety disorders. For example, studies utilizing rodent models exposed to chronic stressors have elucidated the impact of prolonged stress on neural circuits implicated in anxiety (McEwen, 2007). These findings align with observations in humans, where chronic stress is a well-established risk factor for the development of anxiety disorders (Bale, 2006).

Moreover, pharmacological studies in animals have played a crucial role in predicting the efficacy of anxiolytic medications in humans (Holmes, 2003). Drugs targeting specific neurotransmitter systems, identified and tested in animal models, have shown consistent effects in alleviating anxiety symptoms in both preclinical and clinical settings (Nestler & Hyman, 2010). This translational success underscores the shared neurobiological underpinnings of anxiety across species.

Additionally, animal models have contributed substantially to understanding the genetic basis of anxiety susceptibility (Flint & Shifman, 2008). By selectively breeding animals with anxiety-like traits, researchers have identified genes associated with heightened anxiety (NIMH, 2008). These genetic insights have direct relevance to humans, as evidenced by overlapping genetic factors contributing to anxiety disorders in both species (Smoller et al., 2008).

In essence, the translational impact of animal studies extends beyond mere parallels; it actively informs therapeutic strategies and enhances our ability to develop targeted interventions for human anxiety disorders. Recognizing these translational successes reinforces the importance of continued research utilizing comparative psychopathology and animal models in advancing our understanding and treatment of anxiety in humans.

Neurobiological Mechanisms Implicated in Anxiety Cross-Species

The consistency in neurobiological mechanisms implicated in anxiety across species highlights the shared aspects of anxiety-related phenomena in both animals and humans. Similarities in neural circuits, neurotransmitter systems, and molecular pathways underscore the neurobiological consistency of anxiety, fostering a comprehensive understanding of this complex emotion.

Neural circuits play a crucial role in anxiety, and the parallels between animal and human models are evident in the involvement of specific brain regions. The amygdala, prefrontal cortex, and hippocampus consistently emerge as key players in anxiety-related behaviors across various species (LeDoux, 2000; Moreno & González, 2006). Animal studies, particularly in rodents, have provided insights into the intricate interactions within these circuits, offering valuable information that directly translates to our understanding of human anxiety (Likhtik et al., 2014).

The involvement of neurotransmitter systems in anxiety is another area of neurobiological consistency. GABAergic, serotonergic, and noradrenergic systems, among others, exhibit similar modulations in response to stress and anxiety-inducing stimuli across different species (Millan, 2003). Animal models have allowed for precise manipulation of these systems, elucidating their roles in anxiety behaviors and providing data that inform pharmacological interventions in humans (Cryan & Holmes, 2005).

Molecular pathways implicated in anxiety further emphasize cross-species consistency. Common signaling pathways, such as those involving corticotropin-releasing factor (CRF) and neurotrophic factors, demonstrate shared regulatory mechanisms in animals and humans (Duman & Monteggia, 2006). Insights gained from animal studies contribute to our understanding of the molecular underpinnings of anxiety disorders and facilitate the development of targeted therapies.

Overall, the neurobiological consistency in anxiety mechanisms across species, encompassing neural circuits, neurotransmitter systems, and molecular pathways, enriches our understanding of this complex emotional state. Recognizing these similarities allows for a more comprehensive and translational approach to studying and treating anxiety, emphasizing the relevance of comparative psychopathology in advancing mental health research.

Environmental Impact: Parallels Between Environmental Influences on Anxiety in Animals and Humans

In animal models, alterations in environmental conditions, such as exposure to chronic stressors or enriched environments, can significantly modulate anxiety-like behaviors (Fuss et al., 2010; van Praag et al., 2000). For example, rodents exposed to chronic stressors often exhibit increased anxiety-related behaviors, while those in enriched environments, with increased sensory and cognitive stimulation, may show reduced anxiety-like responses.

These findings parallel human experiences, where adverse environmental conditions, such as a history of trauma or chronic stress, are associated with heightened anxiety levels (McLaughlin et al., 2010). Conversely, positive environmental factors, like social support or engaging activities, can contribute to reduced anxiety in humans (Cohen & Wills, 1985).

Furthermore, the impact of early-life environmental exposures on anxiety outcomes is a shared observation across species. Animal studies demonstrate that adverse early-life experiences, such as maternal separation, can contribute to long-lasting changes in anxiety behaviors (Lippmann et al., 2007). Similarly, in humans, early-life adversities have been linked to an increased risk of developing anxiety disorders (Teicher et al., 2003).

Recognizing these parallels highlights the translational significance of environmental manipulations in animal studies. They offer a controlled setting to explore causal relationships between environmental factors and anxiety outcomes, contributing to a deeper understanding of how environmental conditions influence anxiety in both animals and humans.

Overview of Animal Models for Anxiety Disorders

Animal models serve as invaluable tools in unraveling the complexities of anxiety disorders, offering insights into their etiology, mechanisms, and potential treatment avenues. In the following sections, we delve into several established animal models, considering both their strengths and limitations.

Elevated Plus-Maze (EPM)

Strengths: The EPM, proposed by Pellow et al. (1985), assesses rodents' approach-avoidance behavior, providing a reliable measure of anxiety-like responses. An increased duration in the open arms is indicative of reduced anxiety (Pellow et al., 1985).

Limitations: While proficient in capturing unconditioned fear responses, the EPM might fall short in mirroring the chronic and multifaceted nature of clinical anxiety.

Light-Dark Box Test

Strengths: This test, widely employed in anxiety research, evaluates rodents' conflict between the inclination to explore a novel environment and aversion to brightly lit areas. It offers nuanced insights into anxiety-related behaviors (File, 1993).

Limitations: Similar to the EPM, it predominantly focuses on unconditioned fear responses, potentially missing the comprehensive spectrum of clinical anxiety experiences.

Chronic Mild Stress (CMS)

Strengths: Chronic Mild Stress models, as outlined by Willner (2005), subject animals to unpredictable mild stressors, aiming to simulate the chronic stressors contributing to human anxiety disorders. This approach allows researchers to explore stress-induced behaviors (Willner, 2005).

Limitations: While effective in emphasizing stress-related behaviors, CMS may not comprehensively represent the intricate mechanisms underlying anxiety disorders.

Social Defeat Stress

Strengths: This model, discussed by File and Seth (2003), involves exposing animals to social stressors, making it particularly relevant for understanding social anxiety disorders. It addresses the impact of social interactions on anxiety-related behaviors (File & Seth, 2003).

Limitations: It might not fully encapsulate the diverse experiences of social anxiety seen in humans, limiting its applicability.

Fear Conditioning

Strengths: Fear conditioning, a classic model, involves associating a neutral stimulus with an aversive event, allowing researchers to investigate aspects of conditioned fear reminiscent of anxiety disorders (LeDoux, 2000).

Limitations: While proficient in modeling fear responses, it primarily focuses on a specific facet of anxiety, potentially overlooking its multifaceted nature.

Contribution to Understanding Anxiety

- *Etiology*: Animal models enable researchers to explore the interplay of genetic, environmental, and neurobiological factors contributing to anxiety disorders.
- *Mechanisms*: These models provide a platform to dissect the neural circuits, neurotransmitter systems, and molecular pathways intricately involved in anxiety-related phenomena.
- *Treatment Options*: By mimicking key features of anxiety, animal models facilitate the evaluation of potential therapeutic interventions, aiding in drug development.

While acknowledging that no model perfectly mirrors the complexity of human anxiety disorders, the amalgamation of these models enhances our understanding of different facets of anxiety. This fosters translational research that not only benefits animal welfare but also holds promise for advancing treatments for human anxiety disorders.

Functional Aspects of Anxiety Symptoms

One facet is the functional aspect of anxiety symptoms. Within this cognitive domain, heightened vigilance takes center stage. This increased alertness, observed in anxiety, is unpacked to reveal its potential adaptive roots and the evolutionary significance of prioritizing the processing of threatening information (Bateson et al., 2011).

Signal Detection Model in Anxiety Disorders

Moving beyond cognitive nuances, a specific focus can be on anxiety disorders, particularly GAD. GAD can be aptly characterized through the lens of a low threshold in the signal detection model (Bateson et al., 2011; Butler &

Mathews, 1983, 1987; Mathews & MacLeod, 1985). This perspective allows for a coherent understanding of GAD symptoms as extreme manifestations of normal anxiety responses, as outlined in clinical standards such as the DSM-5.

Comprehensive Understanding of GAD Symptoms

There is an interconnectedness of GAD symptoms, including sleep disturbances, tension, and poor concentration. We are establishing a causal link between these symptoms and an individual's markedly low threshold for threat detection (Bateson et al., 2011; Butler & Mathews, 1983, 1987; Mathews & MacLeod, 1985).

Threshold Variation Dynamics

Acknowledging nuanced variations in individuals' thresholds and dynamic shifts within individuals based on evolving life circumstances is important. Likewise, it is crucial to recognize trait-like temperamental differences in threshold positioning and the adaptability of thresholds to changing life situations (Bateson et al., 2011; Butler & Mathews, 1987; Mathews & MacLeod, 1985).

Transformative Façade of Conscious Anticipation in Anxiety

Literature suggests that anxiety as a conscious anticipation of danger is unique to great apes (Belzung & Philippot, 2007). This capacity, linked to autonoetic awareness, is closely tied to the development of the neocortex and its connections with the limbic system and thalamus (Bruce & Neary 1995; Laberge et al., 2006; Monreno & Gonzalez, 2006; Novejarque et al., 2004). The ability to represent oneself and reactions to hypothetical situations is contingent upon strategically activating emotion networks or representations of emotional states, a reflexive capacity shared only by great apes and humans. While other species may have the aptitude to experience anxiety with an anticipation dimension, it may not be conscious or related to the activation of a representation of the situation and its possible consequences. This transformative trend indicates an increase in the complexity of emotional processes and supporting logistical systems from lower to higher levels of the phylum. Higher species retain primitive capabilities while acquiring additional cognitive abilities (Belzung & Philippot, 2007; Bruce & Neary, 1995; Laberge et al., 2006; Monreno & Gonzalez, 2006; Novejarque et al., 2004).

Primitive Aspects in Unicellular Organisms and Nematodes and Anxiety

Even in unicellular organisms like protozoa and ancestral non-segmented worms like nematodes, rudimentary aspects of behavioral responses associated with emotional components are present. These include novelty, pleasantness, goal conduciveness checks, and stress hormones (Belzung & Philippot, 2007; Nieuwenhuys et al., 1998; Northcutt & Kaas, 1995).

In insects, emotional responses are enriched with additional features. This includes an appraisal check for coping potential, specific emotional expressions characterized by postures, vocalizations, and pheromones, and the release of monoamines in response to environmental challenges (Belzung & Philippot, 2007; Nieuwenhuys et al., 1998; Northcutt & Kaas, 1995).

Physiological Responses in Crustaceans and Mollusks

Crustaceans and mollusks demonstrate physiological responses to danger. This distinguishes pure behavioral responses and action tendencies, where physiological indicators may precede behavioral responses (Belzung & Philippot, 2007; Nieuwenhuys et al., 1998; Northcutt & Kaas, 1995; Karten, 1997).

Logistic Systems in Vertebrates

Logistic systems supporting the main facets of human anxiety emerge in vertebrates. Low-order vertebrates possess an autonomic nervous system coordinating physiological responses to stress. Birds display specific responses related to temperature regulation, and mammals, including primates, exhibit a functional amygdala (Belzung & Philippot, 2007; Nieuwenhuys et al., 1998; Northcutt & Kaas, 1995; Karten, 1997).

Sophisticated Emotional Processes in Primates

Primates are characterized by their ability to display specific facial expressions in reaction to danger. They are associated with an important facial musculature. Additionally, primates exhibit sophisticated facets of emotional processes such as autonoetic consciousness, which involves specific connections in prefrontal areas necessary for conscious perception of visceral changes, emotional control, and memory retrieval from past experiences (Belzung & Philippot, 2007; Karten, 1997; Moreno et al., 2005; Nesse & Klaas 1994; Nieuwenhuys et al., 1998; Novejarque et al., 2004; Szekely, 1999).

The coping appraisal check, the diversification of the emotional response (including emotional expression and physiological response), and the capacity for autonoetic awareness emerge as the most relevant dimensions (Eysenck et al., 1991). The ability to assess coping potential distinguishes insects from lower invertebrates, the diversification of the emotional response occurs at higher phylogenetic levels (e.g., facial expressions in monkeys), and autonoetic consciousness appears in great apes (Belzung & Philippot, 2007; Karten, 1997; Nieuwenhuys et al., 1998; Northcutt & Kaas, 1995, Novejarque et al., 2004; Szekely, 1999).

Qualitative Difference Between Human and Animal Anxiety

Research suggests that there is not a qualitative difference between human and animal anxiety. Instead, a clear phylogenetic trend is evident, marked by important steps in the three identified dimensions. The distinctive feature of human anxiety appears to be the well-developed self-awareness capacity, already shared to a lesser extent with great apes. Therefore, the comparative approach proves heuristic for understanding how anxiety varies across phylogeny and for comprehending the underlying processes and logistic systems shaping anxiety (Belzung & Philippot, 2007; Karten, 1997; Lanuza et al., 1997; Nieuwenhuys et al., 1998; Novejarque et al., 2004; Szekely, 1999).

Overall, literature indicates that anxiety as a conscious anticipation of danger is a trait observed exclusively in great apes. This unique capacity, associated with autonoetic awareness, is intricately linked to the development of the neocortex, its connections with the limbic system, and thalamus. Representing oneself and reacting to hypothetical situations depends on the strategic activation of emotion networks, a reflexive capacity shared only by great apes and humans (Belzung & Philippot, 2007).

Therapeutic Implications: Bridging Comparative Approach with Treatment Strategies

The conceptual framework presented in this chapter's discourse offers promising avenues for the development and enhancement of therapeutic interventions. Central to this perspective is the acknowledgment that a person's appraisal of their probability and vulnerability to threats significantly mediates the impact of actual levels of probability and vulnerability. The therapeutic landscape, therefore, can be envisaged as operating on two fronts: altering individuals' objective probability and vulnerability and reshaping their appraisals of these elements (Beck, 1967; Nesse, 2009; Rachman, 1983; Scherer et al., 2001).

Current therapeutic modalities, such as cognitive therapies for anxiety, inherently target the recalibration of either vulnerability or probability, elements integral to the framework. By engaging with individuals' appraisals, these interventions seek to raise the threshold for the manifestation of anxious symptoms. Notably, exposure therapy, a well-established approach for specific phobias, exemplifies how controlled exposure can influence a person's estimate of the probability of a threat, subsequently elevating the threshold for anxious responses (Beck, 1967; Nesse, 2009; Rachman, 1983; Scherer et al., 2001).

Pharmacological interventions for anxiety disorders function by pharmacologically modulating threat detection mechanisms. An intriguing implication from this analysis is that drugs addressing non-anxiety-related symptoms contributing to perceived vulnerability could potentially alleviate anxiety symptoms (Beck, 1967; Nesse, 2009; Rachman, 1983; Scherer et al., 2001). For instance, providing effective analgesia to individuals with chronic pain may inadvertently reduce anxiety symptoms.

A noteworthy facet emphasized by this perspective is the possibility that some individuals experience anxiety as a valid response to realistic appraisals of high probability and vulnerability. In such cases, symptoms of anxiety, though unpleasant, might be adaptive responses to genuine threats (Beck, 1967; Nesse, 2009; Rachman, 1983; Scherer et al., 2001). Consequently, a holistic therapeutic approach necessitates addressing ecological factors, including poverty, economic insecurity, social support deficits, substandard housing, and urban safety concerns. By addressing these ecological determinants, there is potential for population-level benefits, leading to reduced rates of anxiety across communities. This underscores the importance of integrating ecological considerations alongside cognitive interventions in the broader spectrum of mental health strategies.

Conclusion

This book chapter, "*Beyond the Basics of Anxiety Disorders: A Comparative Psychopathology Perspective*" aims to provide a comprehensive and in-depth exploration of anxiety disorders, beyond the fundamental understanding. The comprehensive exploration of anxiety in this discourse sheds light on its pervasive impact, emphasizing the need for nuanced therapeutic interventions.

The incorporation of a comparative approach across species highlights the shared evolutionary purpose of anxiety, while the examination of Generalized Anxiety Disorder through the signal detection model provides a coherent framework for understanding its manifestations. Evolutionary insights, spanning from unicellular organisms to primates, showcase the adaptive nature of ALR. The acknowledgment of individual variations in threshold dynamics and the transformative trend of conscious anticipation in great apes underscores the complexity of emotional processes across phylogeny.

Therapeutically, the proposed framework aligns with current modalities, urging a focus on both objective alterations and individuals' appraisals. Recognizing anxiety as a potentially valid response to genuine threat calls for a holistic approach that addresses ecological factors, ultimately contributing to population-level benefits and reduced anxiety rates across communities. By adopting a comparative psychopathology approach, the chapter highlights the value of studying anxiety-related behaviors in nonhuman animals and possible treatment.

References

American Psychiatric Association. (2013). *Diagnostic and Statistical Manual of Mental Disorders* (5th ed.). Arlington, VA: American Psychiatric Publishing.

Bale, T. L. (2006). Stress sensitivity and the development of affective disorders. *Hormones and Behavior*, *50*(4), 529–533.

Bateson, M., Brilot, B., & Nettle, D. (2011). Anxiety: An evolutionary approach. *Canadian Journal of Psychiatry*, *56*(12), 707–715.

Beck, A. T. (1967). *Depression*. New York: Hoeber Medical Division.

Belzung, C., & Philippot, P. (2007). Anxiety from a phylogenetic perspective: Is there a qualitative difference between human and animal anxiety? *Neural Plasticity*, *30*(2),1–17. https://doi.org/10.1155/2007/59676

Brilot, B. O., Asher, L., & Bateson, M. (2010). Stereotyping starlings are more 'pessimistic'. *Animal Cognition*, *13*(5), 721–731.

Bruce, L. L., & Neary, T. J. (1995). The limbic system of tetrapods: A comparative analysis of cortical and amygdalar populations. *Brain, Behavior and Evolution*, *46*(4–5), 224–234.

Burman, O. H. P., Parker, R. M. A., Paul, E. S., et al. (2009). Anxiety-induced cognitive bias in non-human animals. *Physiology & Behavior*, *98*(3), 345–350.

Butler, G., & Mathews, A. (1983). Cognitive processes in anxiety. *Advances in Behaviour Research and Therapy*, *5*(1), 51–62.

Butler, G., & Mathews, A. (1987). Anticipatory anxiety and risk perception. *Cognitive Therapy Research*, *11*(5), 551–565.

Cohen, S., & Wills, T. A. (1985). Stress, social support, and the buffering hypothesis. *Psychological Bulletin*, *98*(2), 310.

Cryan, J. F., & Holmes, A. (2005). The ascent of mouse: Advances in modelling human depression and anxiety. *Nature Reviews Drug Discovery*, *4*(9), 775–790.

Duman, R. S., & Monteggia, L. M. (2006). A neurotrophic model for stress-related mood disorders. *Biological Psychiatry*, *59*(12), 1116–1127.

Eysenck, M. W., Mogg, K., May, J., et al. (1991). Bias in interpretation of ambiguous sentences related to threat in anxiety. *Journal of Abnormal Psychology*, *100*(2), 144–150.

File, S. E. (1993). The use of social interaction as a method for detecting anxiolytic activity of chlordiazepoxide-like drugs. *Journal of Neuroscience Methods*, *38*(3), 169–174.

File, S. E., & Seth, P. (2003). A review of 25 years of the social interaction test. *European Journal of Pharmacology*, *463*(1–3), 35–53.

Flint, J., & Shifman, S. (2008). Animal models of psychiatric disease. *Current Opinion in Genetics & Development*, *18*(3), 235–240. https://doi.org/10.1016/j.gde.2008.07.002

Fuss, J., Ben Abdallah, N. M. B., Hensley, F. W., Weber, K. J., Hellweg, R., & Gass, P. (2010). Deletion of running-induced hippocampal neurogenesis by irradiation prevents the development of an anxious phenotype in mice. *PLoS ONE*, *5*(9), e12769.

Griebel, G., Simiand, J., Serradeil-Le Gal, C., Wagnon, J., Pascal, M., Scatton, B., & Soubrie, P. (2002). Anxiolytic-and antidepressant-like effects of the non-peptide vasopressin V1b receptor antagonist, SSR149415, suggest an innovative approach for the treatment of stress-related disorders. *Proceedings of the National Academy of Sciences*, *99*(9), 6370–6375.

Holmes, A. (2003). Targeted gene mutation approaches to the study of anxiety-like behavior in mice. *Neuroscience & Biobehavioral Reviews*, *27*(3), 273–289.

Karten, H. J. (1997). Evolutionary developmental biology meets the brain: The origins of mammalian cortex. *Proceedings of the National Academy of Sciences of the United States of America, 94*(7), 2800–2804.

Kessler, R. C., Chiu, W. T., Demler, O., et al. (2005). Prevalence, severity, and comorbidity of 12-month DSM-IV disorders in the National Comorbidity Survey Replication. *Archives of General Psychiatry, 62,* 617–627.

Laberge, F., Muhlenbrock-Lenter, S., Grunwald, W., & Roth, G. (2006). Evolution of the amygdala: New insights from studies in amphibians. *Brain, Behavior and Evolution, 67*(4), 177–187.

Lanuza, E., Font, C., Martínez-Marcos, A., & Martínez-García, F. (1997). Amygdalo-hypothalamic projections in the lizard Podarcis hispanica: A combined anterograde and retrograde tracing study. *Journal of Comparative Neurology, 384*(4), 537–555.

LeDoux, J. E. (2000). Emotion circuits in the brain. *Annual Review of Neuroscience, 23*(1), 155–184.

Likhtik, E., Stujenske, J. M., Topiwala, M. A., Harris, A. Z., & Gordon, J. A. (2014). Prefrontal entrainment of amygdala activity signals safety in learned fear and innate anxiety. *Nature Neuroscience, 17*(1), 106–113.

Lippmann, M., Bress, A., Nemeroff, C. B., Plotsky, P. M., & Monteggia, L. M. (2007). Long-term behavioural and molecular alterations associated with maternal separation in rats. *European Journal of Neuroscience, 25*(10), 3091–3098.

Mateo, J. M. (2007). Ecological and hormonal correlates of antipredator behavior in adult Belding's ground squirrels (*Spermophilus beldingi*). *Behavioral Ecology and Sociobiology, 62*(1), 37–49.

Mathews, A., & MacLeod, C. (1985). Selective processing of threat cues in anxiety states. *Behaviour Research and Therapy, 23*(5), 563–569. https://doi.org/10.1016/0005-7967(85)90104-4

McEwen, B. S. (2007). Physiology and neurobiology of stress and adaptation: Central role of the brain. *Physiological Reviews, 87*(3), 873–904.

McLaughlin, K. A., Kubzansky, L. D., Dunn, E. C., Waldinger, R., Vaillant, G., & Koenen, K. C. (2010). Childhood social environment, emotional reactivity to stress, and mood and anxiety disorders across the life course. *Depression and Anxiety, 27*(12), 1087–1094.

Millan, M. J. (2003). The neurobiology and control of anxious states. *Progress in Neurobiology, 70*(2), 83–244.

Moreno, N., & González, A. (2006). The common organization of the amygdaloid complex in tetrapods: New concepts based on developmental, hodological and neurochemical data in anuran amphibians. *Progress in Neurobiology, 78*(2), 61–90.

Moreno, N., Morona, R., López, J. M., Muñoz, M., & González, A. (2005). Lateral and medial amygdala of anuran amphibians and their relation to olfactory and vomeronasal information. *Brain Research Bulletin, 66*(4–6), 332–336.

National Institute of Mental Health (NIMH). (2008). Animal research on anxiety-like behavior. Retrieved from https://www.nimh.nih.gov/health/topics/animal-research-on-anxiety-like-behavior/index.shtml

Nesse, R. M., & Klaas, R. (1994). Risk perception by patients with anxiety disorders. *Journal of Nervous and Mental Disease, 182,* 465–470.

Nesse, R. M. (2009). Explaining depression: Neuroscience is not enough, evolution is essential. *Understanding Depression: A translational Approach, 17*–35.

Nestler, E. J., & Hyman, S. E. (2010). Animal models of neuropsychiatric disorders. *Nature Neuroscience, 13*(10), 1161–1169.

Nieuwenhuys, R., ten Donkelaar, H. J., & Nicholson, C. (1998). *The Central Nervous System of Vertebrates*. Berlin, Germany: Springer.

Northcutt, R. G., & Kaas, J. H. (1995). The emergence and evolution of mammalian neocortex. *Trends in Neurosciences, 18*(9), 373–379.

Novejarque, A., Lanuza, E., & Martínez-García, F. (2004). Amygdalostriatal projections in reptiles: A tract-tracing study in the lizard Podarcis hispanica. *Journal of Comparative Neurology, 479*(3), 287–308.

Pellow, S., Chopin, P., Eddy, P., Mittleman, G., Rawlins, J., & File, S. E. (1985). Validation of open: Closed arm entries in an elevated plus-maze as a measure of anxiety in the rat. *Journal of Neuroscience Methods, 14*(3), 149–167.

Rachman, S. (1983). The modification of agoraphobic avoidance behaviour: some fresh possibilities. *Behaviour Research and Therapy, 21*(5), 567–574.

Santarelli, L., Saxe, M., Gross, C., Surget, A., Battaglia, F., Dulawa, S., ... & Hen, R. (2003). Requirement of hippocampal neurogenesis for the behavioral effects of antidepressants. *Science, 301*(5634), 805–809.

Scherer, K. R., Schorr, A., & Johnstone, T. (Eds.). (2001). *Appraisal processes in emotion: Theory, methods, research*. Oxford University Press.

Smoller, J. W., Gardner-Schuster, E., Covino, J. M., & The Bipolar Disorder Genome Study Consortium. (2008). The genetic basis of panic and phobic anxiety disorders. *American Journal of Medical Genetics Part C: Seminars in Medical Genetics, 148*(2), 118–126.

Stein, D. J., Scott, K. M., de Jonge, P., et al. (2017). Epidemiology of anxiety disorders: From surveys to nosology and back. *Dialogues in Clinical Neuroscience, 19*, 127–136.

Székely, A. D. (1999). The avian hippocampal formation: Subdivisions and connectivity. *Behavioural Brain Research, 98*(2), 219–225.

Teicher, M. H., Andersen, S. L., Polcari, A., Anderson, C. M., Navalta, C. P., & Kim, D. M. (2003). The neurobiological consequences of early stress and childhood maltreatment. *Neuroscience & Biobehavioral Reviews, 27*(1–2), 33–44.

van Praag, H., Kempermann, G., & Gage, F. H. (2000). Neural consequences of environmental enrichment. *Nature Reviews Neuroscience, 1*(3), 191–198.

Willner, P. (2005). Chronic mild stress (CMS) revisited: Consistency and behavioural-neurobiological concordance in the effects of CMS. *Neuropsychobiology, 52*(2), 90–110.

5 Comparative Psychopathology and Repetitive Behaviors

Introduction

Comparative psychopathology offers a path to study different symptoms that occur across various psychological disorders. Depression and anxiety are two different categories in the *DSM-5*, but there are many crossovers between the two categories. Anxiety often occurs in depression (Zimmerman et al., 2019), and depression is common for individuals with anxiety disorders (Haller et al., 2021). Similarly, heavy substance use occurs in many other psychiatric disorders (Helle et al., 2020), and aggression is associated with multiple mood disorders (Rice et al., 2022).

In the psychopathology world, instead, amusing terms are used to debate between those who focus more on the similarities between what might seem like different conditions and those who focus on overlapping other conditions (Goodwin, 2015). This debate is called one between the "lumpers" (those focused on similarities) and the "splitters" (those focused on overlap). *DSM-5* is more in the "splitter" category, although its focus does change for certain categories. Similarly, comparative psychology is most likely considered in the "lumper" category, although this is likely not a pure classification, and the emphasis could change in some areas.

In the article summarizing the "lumpers" and "splitters" debate, Goodwin summarizes one of the limitations presently associated with diagnoses and accounting for some of the grouping of symptoms that may not always be warranted. Here is the summary statement:

> Therefore, a diagnosis of major depression, an anxiety disorder, or OCD may make perfect sense in terms of the primary symptoms of which the patient complains and on which a differentiated diagnosis is based, yet there may well be a common experience of anxiety and even dysphoria across the conditions, and of course recourse to the same drug or choice of drugs for treatment.

DOI: 10.4324/9781003408918-6

This statement comes from a neuroscience journal, so the emphasis on medication (rather than giving equal consideration to psychotherapy) is to be expected. When disregarding that emphasis, notice how the focus is on the limitations that verbal language brings to the understanding of psychopathology. Goodwin brings up here the degree to which treating and studying psychological disorders can be limited by a reliance on what the human experiencing the symptoms reports.

Relying on verbal self-reports about psychological symptoms is a criticism that has been lobbed against current approaches to psychopathology. This criticism has been directed toward the DSM-5 (Chmielewski et al., 2015; Ganellen, 2014). The weaknesses of relying on self-reports in clinical practice and research have been criticized in symposia addressing mental health research and care (Garcia & Gustavson, 1997). There are weak correlations between what people report as symptoms and what they show through observable behaviors (Dang et al., 2020; Keefer, 2015).

One of the benefits of comparative psychology is that it removes verbal language as a means by which the cause of symptoms is defined. Comparative psychopathology considers research across species, but verbal language is taken out of the equation. Behavioral patterns must be assessed based on what is observed rather than what the individual says is the problem. Studying nonhuman animals and human animals means explaining behaviors cannot be focused on whether the person states verbally that they feel "anxious" or "depressed." When words are removed as a possible source of defining what contributes to an individual's behavior, thus meaning that behaviors are studied only by objective observations, there is more room to consider similarities across different conditions. In other words, symptoms of conditions like depression and anxiety can be studied without considering whether the person uses the words "depression" or "anxiety" to describe what is happening.

Comparative psychopathology allows for the study of psychological disorders from a much more objective and behavioral perspective than other approaches. Symptoms and contributing factors are studied without relying on asking the individual what they are experiencing. There is no need to consider subjective experience, which is a benefit because of how subjective experiences can be influenced. Similarities between anxiety and depression can be viewed without being influenced by whether the individual describes themselves as "nervous" (more associated with anxiety disorders) or "sad" (more related to depressive disorders). It is even possible that a comprehensive field of comparative psychopathology could show that the similarities of behaviors considered separate from what individuals state about their subjective experiences could indicate that diagnostic categories now regarded as distinct could be the same.

Comparative psychopathology represents an approach to understanding psychopathology that removes self-report and other subjective constructs when defining and understanding psychopathology. Verbal self-reports do not play a major role in comparative psychopathology because their research basis relies on research where verbal speech is not emphasized (since many subjects studied are nonhumans and do not rely on verbal speech). As such, it allows for consideration of behaviors and overt symptoms that present across disorders without relying on verbal statements that can delineate different conditions (e.g., "I feel depressed," "My nerves get so bad I can't shut off my negative thoughts"). When individuals try to describe what they are feeling or why they are feeling a certain way, it can lead to a mislabeling of symptoms and behaviors relating to what the individual reports. Individuals are often poor judges of the source of their difficulties, and removing their subjective conclusions can help strengthen the understanding of what is happening with psychological symptoms.

Verbal speech is not ignored in comparative psychopathology; it is just not emphasized. When verbal speech is considered, it is regarded as a behavior that follows the rules of other behaviors. It is observed and measured as a behavior. This has a long history within the behavioral analysis field, where verbal behavior among humans has been considered to follow similar rules to other overt behaviors (Carroll, 1944; McGuigan, 1970; Horne & Lowe, 1997). From a behavioral perspective, language is like every other behavior and follows the same rules of behavior (LaFrance & Tarbox, 2020). Words people use to follow the same rules as other behaviors. They exist and are considered alongside other behaviors. Similarly, thoughts and thinking are also considered as internal or "covert" behaviors (Feng & Wang, 2022; Kelly & Kelly, 2022; Tichenor & Yaruss, 2021). Data about these covert behaviors are gathered from the words people use to describe those experiences (which are not emphasized in this approach and are treated as observable behaviors following the same rules as other behaviors).

As discussed in this chapter so far, comparative psychopathology focuses on observable symptoms that occur across different psychological disorders and different psychological constructs (e.g., anxiety). This offers a new approach that helps discuss groups of disorders together and discuss symptoms in more dimensional rather than categorical ways. Symptoms are discussed in terms of how they are common across different disorders rather than how they are different. Empirical research shows evidence for understanding the cause of these observable symptoms common across various disorders. In this way, comparative psychopathology offers a path for practitioners to "treat the source, not the symptoms" (Hale & Hale, 2010).

A brief review is in order before discussing one of these symptoms that overlap between diagnoses. The previous chapters show evidence of a need for a new way of defining psychopathology. This is because current methods focus too much on one area of functioning, primarily related to neurology or medical biology, and less on the whole individual. There also is a need for psychopathology understanding that incorporates clinical, neurological, and medical research and basic, observational, and experimental research across all domains. Each of these issues can be addressed with an approach to understanding psychopathology that emphasizes comparative psychology, which we call comparative psychopathology.

In the material covered in this chapter, we see that comparative psychopathology also allows for more consideration of observable symptoms that crossover between different diagnoses. This approach to psychopathology falls more in the "lumper" category than the "splitter category." This would help keep the study of psychopathology more consistent with the research showing the similarities between multiple diagnoses. It also provides an opportunity to lessen the amount of therapeutic and medical approaches that all seem to have the same approach but claim to target different conditions. This is what Nuttgens (2023) termed "interventitive doppelgangers". Utilizing an approach to understanding psychopathology that emphasizes similarities could help address the rapidly increasing problem of polypharmacy (i.e., using multiple medications for the same problems patients report) in psychiatry (Kukreja et al., 2023).

Repetitive Behaviors Across Different Diagnoses

This chapter addresses one behavioral symptom that occurs across a number of different psychological disorders: repetitive behaviors. Several diagnostic categories have repetitive behaviors as a symptom. Repetitive negative self-statements are common symptoms across many different diagnoses (Ehring & Watkins, 2008; Watkins & Roberts, 2020). Negative self-statements that a person says to themselves constantly, also called "rumination," are a major factor in depressive disorders (Tackman et al., 2019; Taylor & Snyder, 2021)). Anxiety disorders also have repetitive negative self-statements (Mursaleen, 2023). Repetitive motor behaviors and repetitive verbal statements are a required symptom for a *DSM-5* diagnosis of autism (Wiggens et al., 2019). These types of repeating behaviors are essentially the defining characteristic of obsessive-compulsive disorder (Szejko & Müller-Vahl, 2021; Oliveira et al., 2019). Repetitive negative thinking about self and the world is a common behavioral characteristic of schizophrenia and other psychotic disorders (Zagaria et al., 2023). Certain forms of addiction are also seen as having repetitive behaviors as a major characteristic (Reichert et al., 2021).

There is evidence from psychotherapy literature supporting the consideration of repetitive negative thoughts as the same as other repetitive behaviors. Repetitive self-statements are seen in cognitive therapy as internal behaviors that occur across a number of psychological disorders (Beck, 1991; Feldhaus et al., 2020). Rumination, seen this way, is a habit that can be addressed using cognitive-behavioral therapy approaches to address other habits (Watkins, 2018). Behavior therapy approaches like Acceptance and Commitment Therapy (ACT) use the same behavioral constructs to explain ruminative thoughts as are used for other behaviors (Dereix-Calonge et al., 2019; Mansueto et al., 2021; Ruiz et al., 2018). Applied behavior analysis discusses ruminative thoughts like other repetitive behaviors (Luiselli, 2015; Migan-Gandonou & Leon, 2020; Woods et al., 2013). Repetitive negative thinking associated with both anxiety and depression is discussed in the behavior therapy literature as following the same constructs as other behaviors (Monteregge et al., 2020; Spinhoven et al., 2018).

Repetitive behaviors make up a significant part of psychological behaviors. What tends to happen in most psychological disorders is that the individual gets caught in a pattern of engaging in behaviors repeatedly that are unhealthy and problematic. The individual develops what is called a habit where they repeatedly engage in behaviors that are not helpful and cause more problems for themselves and other people around them. It is often the person's desire to break that habit, yet the habit of incorporating these repetitive behaviors becomes something that the person cannot break. Some examples of repetitive behaviors that make up psychological disorders include the following:

- A person repeatedly calls themselves a "loser" and finds evidence in multiple areas of their lives where they have not reached what they believed to be their potential (depressive disorder).
- A teenager flaps their arms frequently throughout the day in a manner very disruptive to their classes and other people around them (autism).
- A person interrupts their days multiple times because they believe they have to turn a doorknob to the right 42 times in a row or else something terrible will happen to someone they love (obsessive-compulsive disorder)
- A person repeatedly tells themselves that people are watching them and that they need to be on the lookout for spies; they continue this behavior even in the absence of any objective evidence (schizophrenic disorders)
- A person paces up and down the hallway at work for no reason other than they are feeling restless and nervous (anxiety disorder)
- A person cannot turn off their social media feed and stop looking at it even though they have not seen anything particularly interesting on it for days (digital media addiction)

Repetitive Behaviors Across the Animal World

Repetitive behaviors are common in the animal world. Many are part of normal functioning out in the wild. Repeatedly performed action patterns are common among animals as a means of survival and adjusting to their environments. These include the repetitive behaviors for building nests and following repetitive paths for collecting food. Animals like birds, rats, lions, prairie dogs, and squirrels all engage in these types of behaviors and must engage in them to survive. Behavioral patterns like this are considered normal and typically have some purpose. Comparative psychology research goes back to the discussed adaptive roles for repetitive behaviors as they helped young humans and animals learn about their environment and how to function in it.

Then, there are repetitive behaviors considered abnormal. These include pacing behaviors among certain birds, jumping in mice, rocking behaviors in certain primates, and self-injurious behaviors in certain monkeys (Langen et al., 2011a, 2011b). Behaviors like these are repetitive, often many times, and serve no apparent purpose. They may start as behaviors with some specific purpose, but the frequency and duration with which they repeat serve no apparent purpose and no clear benefit for the individual.

It is the fact that these repetitive behaviors occur for no apparent reason and no clear benefit that makes them of particular interest to the study of psychopathology. Whether it is repetitive negative self-statements made by a person with depression or repetition of a movie quote by someone with autism, it is the repetition that is the most noteworthy pathological component. A person stating that they had failed in one business attempt may be understandable, or a person repeating a movie quote might be interesting, but engaging in these behaviors frequently and over extended periods becomes problematic.

Abnormal repetitive behaviors occur among humans and nonhuman animals due to genetic, biochemical, and environmental factors. Genetic factors that cause abnormal repetitive behaviors include the deletion of the DLG2 gene (Yoo et al., 2020). Variations of the CRISPR/Cas9 genome have also been shown to be involved (Horie et al., 2019). KCTD12 genomes were found to have significant associations with rumination (Eslari et al., 2019) along with the more specific gene KCNH3 (Eslari et al., 2021).

Neurochemical factors impacting repetitive behaviors include postnatal exposure to valproic acid (Eissa et al., 2019). Excessive levels of the neurotransmitter glutamate are strongly associated with abnormal repetitive behaviors (Katz et al., 2019). Neurological factors include reduced activity of the hippocampus (Amodeo et al., 2019). Disruptions in connections between the cerebellum and prefrontal cortex are related to repetitive behaviors (Jacobs et al., 2020; Kelly et al., 2020). Zhang et al. (2020) showed support that both the hippocampus and prefrontal cortex regions were involved with repetitive behaviors associated with negative rumination.

Tonna et al. (2020) presented a path by which genetic, neurochemical, and environmental factors interact to cause and maintain abnormal repetitive behaviors. Certain repetitive behaviors are genetically programmed for certain species. These typically serve some means by which the species is helped to survive in their environment. In the comparative psychology literature, this is known as "exaptations." As the individual of a species develops, normal neurochemical processes along with social learning led to further development and strengthening of these behaviors. The unpredictability of environments often leads to changes in how repetitive these behaviors become. Even if certain behaviors tend to occur to manage the typical environment an individual of a species may have to maneuver, it is rarely the case that the actual environments meet the expectations of what is considered typical. Behaviors genetically or neurochemically programmed for individuals taught to individuals may become more repetitive and ritualistic in more unpredictable environments.

From a comparative psychopathological perspective, it is interesting that the Tonna article addresses repetitive behaviors, which the authors call "ritualized" behaviors, through the "four questions" important to comparative psychology. The famous Dutch Zoologist Niko Tinbergen initially presented these questions in his famous 1963 paper "On The Aims and Methods of Ethology." Then, the translation from German was discussed in Taborsky (2014). The first two questions relate to what processes contribute to the development of a biological trait and what biological mechanisms and structures serve to make that trait work to accomplish its function. Then, the following two questions relate to how historically the trait has helped the species survive and what factors help the individual adapt to its unique environment. All four questions are essential for understanding any behavior. The fourth question strongly relates to why one individual may have an abnormal degree of repetition or ritualization of otherwise adaptive behaviors.

Although neurological and genetic factors may be the main reason these repetitive behaviors start, environmental factors are what tend to increase their severity. Isolation, including that associated with confinement, is one environmental factor related to abnormal repetitive behaviors. Repetitive behaviors represent the most frequently observed pathological behaviors found in animals living in confined spaces (Gandhi & Lee, 2021; Lewis et al., 2007). Once the restrictions associated with confinement are reduced, the frequency and duration of repetitive behaviors tend also to decrease (Yoo et al., 2020).

Harry Harlow is credited with some of the earliest work on abnormal repetitive behaviors in animal species. His work on monkeys raised in isolation (Harlow & Harlow, 1962; Harlow & Suomi, 1971; Suomi et al., 1970) showed that repetitive behaviors that were deemed depressive increased significantly with these monkeys, along with significant decreases in exploratory behaviors. These repetitive behaviors considered depressive included huddling behaviors. Monkeys raised during their earliest days in isolation showed a strong tendency to engage in the same behavior, huddling, that would be used as a defense against predators. Notice how these fits in with the social competition theory discussed in an earlier chapter, where depressive behaviors occur as a defense against facing threats from a stronger potential adversary.

Stress is another environmental factor that tends to increase repetitive behaviors. Experiencing increased stress tends to increase repetitive behaviors, but the behaviors themselves are not caused by anxiety (Lustberg et al., 2020; Lustberg et al., 2022). This is consistent with findings that treatments for decreasing stress can help reduce repetitive behaviors of obsessive-compulsive disorders along with those associated with autism and Tourette's Disorder. Stress, most likely to cause abnormal repetitive behaviors, is associated with major changes in the animal's environment (Sulkama et al., 2022). These changes can include physiological changes, low levels of exercise, increased isolation, family changes, and neurological injuries.

How Comparative Psychopathology Helps Advance Understanding of Repetitive Behaviors

Reviews of comparative psychology literature show that several genetic and neurochemical factors contribute to repetitive behaviors across animal species. Environmental factors shown to impact these behaviors are isolation and stress. These are shown to be contributing factors to behaviors that individuals repeat and that, although on a less frequent and/or shorter basis, may have important purpose, have no clear purpose or benefit to the individual if they occur frequently over relatively long periods.

It is interesting to consider what these findings show about the repetitive behaviors associated with psychological disorders. Isolation is defined as objectively being alone and is differentiated from loneliness, defined as feeling alone. It is interesting here to remember that one of the benefits of comparative psychology research is that it focuses mainly on objective behaviors and does not rely on what the individual reports about how they are feeling. Research on repetitive behaviors from this perspective shows the impact of an individual being without other social interaction separate from whether the individual describes themselves as feeling "lonely."

Social isolation is a major factor in an increased amount of repetitive motor behaviors in autism (Martínez-González et al., 2022). One of the main behavioral symptoms of autism is impaired social behaviors, and this often leads to social isolation being a problem. Studies show not only that social isolation is a problem associated with increased repetitive behaviors but also that interventions designed to improve social skills and increase positive social interactions tend to decrease repetitive motor behaviors.

Isolation increased significantly during the COVID-19 pandemic, providing a unique opportunity to study the impact of isolation on repetitive behaviors. It was a unique research opportunity because it allowed for studying isolation rather than loneliness since the regulations required people to stay alone. Following these regulations meant people spent more time alone, even if they would not have used the term "lonely" to describe how they felt. Repetitive negative thinking about hopelessness was found to increase significantly as a means by which anxiety increased during the pandemic (Dos Santos et al., 2021; Wilkialis et al., 2021; Zorzo, Méndez-López et al., 2019).

Compulsive hair-pulling (trichotillomania) and skin-picking, both disorders falling under the "Obsessive-Compulsive Disorders" category of DSM- 5, were found to increase significantly in relation to increased social isolation (Alhetheli et al., 2022). Repetitive paranoid thoughts were found to increase significantly both in frequency and severity with increased social isolation (Fett et al., 2022).

Fighting against social isolation is seen as having an evolutionary benefit as it protects the individual from being alone in fights against predators and starvation. As a subjective feeling, loneliness is seen as having an impact as it is an internal warning against social isolation. When loneliness is studied from this perspective, primarily in the context of its relation to social isolation, research shows a strong connection between social isolation, feelings of loneliness (serving as a trigger that social isolation is occurring), and the repetitive negative thoughts associated with depression (Cacioppo et al., 2014; Goosens et al., 2015; Heatley et al., 2020; Keller et al., 2023; Spithoven et al., 2019).

Studying stress as a variable is more difficult than studying isolation. Primarily, this is because there are different definitions of stress. As Levine (1985) noted, the different definitions can often be paradoxical; agitated animals and immobile animals could both be considered "stressed". In comparative psychology literature, stress is defined as the individual animal's response to a hostile environment. It is, in a somewhat more technical manner, the individual's "external body forces used to displace homeostasis (Stott,1981). It has also been described as "the inability of an animal to cope with its environment" (Dobson & Smith, 2000).

Stress can best be defined as when the environmental demands imposed exceed an organism's ability to adapt (Koolhaas et al., 2017). This relatively recent definition incorporates most of the main definitions used until now (McCarty, 2020). Stress also typically involves physiological responses from the whole body. Measurements of stress include multiple measures of physiological factors and evidence of how the organism responds to environmental demands.

Notice again how the definition of stress here, which fits nicely into the study of comparative psychopathology due to how it is based on comparative psychology research, focuses on objectively observable data and not subjective self-reports. Evidence of an individual showing signs of being overwhelmed by environmental demands can be observed, separate from what the individual reports verbally. These methods move beyond an emphasis on gauging any sort of subjective material like how the person is "feeling" (Epel et al., 2018).

Similar to isolation, stress as an objective, measurable variable (measured through behaviors, blood pressure, physiological responses, eye dilation, breathing patterns, and body posture) has been associated with several psychological disorders. One example of this is body posture, which can be seen in terms of how an individual stands and adjusts their body (Bergström et al., 2016). Another example of an objective measure of stress from a physiological direction is significantly decreased white blood cell counts (Puta et al., 2018).

Defined in this objective way, stress is significantly related to a number of psychological disorders and, specifically, to the repetitive behaviors associated with those disorders. Repetitive negative thinking and rumination are significantly associated with increased stress in depressive disorders (Hasegawa et al., 2023; Mezo & Baker, 2012). Stress has been found to be significantly associated with repetitive and stereotyped behaviors (e.g., repetitive pacing) in psychotic disorders like schizophrenia (Caponnetto et al., 2021; Dahlen et al., 2021). Repetitive and stereotyped behaviors significantly increase in individuals with autism when subject to increased stress (Nadeem et al., 2019; Williams et al., 2021). Behaviors repeated frequently are also associated with increased observable signs of stress for individuals with obsessive-compulsive disorders (Kracker Imthon et al., 2020; Santore et al., 2020). Repetitive negative statements about self and the world are also related to increased stress in anxiety disorders (Aziziaram & Basharpoor, 2020; Cook et al., 2019).

Repetitive Behaviors and Veterinary Psychiatry

Repetitive behaviors make up a large part of symptomology associated with psychopathology in nonhuman animals. Tail-chasing in dogs can become so repetitive that it presents pathological problems (d'Angelo et al., 2022). Similarly, repetitive and loud barking for no clear reason is also a common reflection of anxiety in dogs (Dinwoodie et al., 2019; Yamada et al., 2019). Unusually high amounts of repetitive light play are associated with compulsive behavior disorders in cats (Kogan & Grigg, 2021). Repetitive behaviors also have been identified as a common behavior issue associated with animals experiencing stress related to physical pain (Mills et al., 2020). Rats and mice are also animals who show evidence of anxiety, measured using behavioral observation and physiological data through repetitive behaviors (Perez Garcia et al., 2021).

Behavioral pathology in nonhuman animals also often involves repetitive avoidance of social situations. This sort of behavioral inhibition is evident across problems many nonhuman primates face (Capitanio, 2018). It is also interesting that behavioral instruments assess nonhuman personality traits, including repetitive behaviors. This includes the "Elephant Behavior Index" used at large animal parks, including Disney's Animal Kingdon (Grand et al., 2012). Among other behavior types, behavioral measures addressing repetitive behaviors indicative of animal psychopathology have been used with animals such as pigs, sheep, and goats (Kirk & Ramsden, 2018). Repetitive oral behaviors have been shown through such methods to be associated with stress related to food insufficiency (Lawrence & Terlouw, 1993; Schouten, Rushen & De Passillé, 1991). Stress related to environmental factors is significantly related to repetitive explanatory behaviors in reptiles that occur for no clear purpose (Bashaw et al., 2016).

As shown earlier in this chapter, stress and isolation also are significantly associated with increased evidence of psychopathology in nonhuman animals. Research showing how observable and measurable data is associated with human psychological disorders often comes from comparative psychology research. That same research supports that stress and isolation play major roles in understanding pathological symptoms among nonhuman animals. Understanding the role of stresses and isolation in nonhuman animal pathological behaviors offers considerable benefit for advancing veterinary psychiatry. This is particularly the case with domesticated animals. For decades, zoos were a prime example of how isolation impacted nonhuman animals (Maple, 2007). Even today, there is much debate that even the more open architecture of zoos still hurts animals. Cages for domesticated animals also cause isolation, and prolonged caging risks pathological responses. Pet owners often keep domesticated dogs and cats in cages for their safety and the household's protection. It is beneficial to consider what sort of psychological impact this common approach to pet ownership might have.

Just the minimal sample of the vast amount of research that exists related to pathological behaviors in nonhuman animals shows that comparative psychopathology offers benefits not just to studying human pathology but also nonhuman pathology. Veterinary psychiatry is a relatively new field in terms of being a formal discipline, and its newness means that there has not been time to incorporate all the relevant information across the comparative psychology field. Developing an approach to studying and understanding nonhuman psychopathology requires one that does not require verbal speech or self-assessment. Comparative psychopathology offers this approach and is a method that could as comfortably fit in veterinary psychiatry as it would in human psychiatry.

There is a whole field of nonhuman psychopathology that needs to be advanced if humans are going to be fair and moral in their treatment of their nonhuman counterparts. Behaviors reflect multiple pathologies among individual organisms who cannot speak for themselves. These include the dogs, cats, reptiles, and birds that humans keep as pets. Animals that provide the wool we wear and milk we treat need to be treated humanely, including psychological health considerations. This goes as well with the animals (e.g., elephants, tigers, and lions) that provide entertainment through zoos and circuses until recently. There even needs to be consideration of the psychological well-being of animals that eventually will become the food people eat. Although these animals will meet their end at the hands of humans, those same humans have a moral responsibility to make sure their psychological well-being is maintained while under their care.

Summary

Throughout this book, we have presented comparative psychopathology as a new way of defining the study of psychological disorders. One approach to this difference would be to redefine how specific psychological disorders and psychological constructs are defined. Depression and anxiety are two examples of psychological disorder types, and psychological constructs can be redefined differently using an approach that emphasizes experimental and observational research along with clinical and medical research. Using scientific research across all the psychological fields, rather than just those related to the clinical fields, gives a much more comprehensive understanding of those disorders and constructs.

In this chapter, we have already built on the material presented in terms of what comparative psychopathology offers by looking more directly at how comparative psychopathology can be a different way of defining psychological disorders. Indeed, the category of repetitive behaviors is one that is emphasized more, with certain psychological disorders. autism being a clear example, but what we have seen throughout this chapter is that repetitive behaviors are a major aspect of a number of different psychological disorders. This chapter specifically looked at repetitive behaviors (including repetitive negative thoughts and rumination as nonverbal repetitive behaviors that follow the same rules as objective behaviors) as a major aspect of depression, anxiety, obsessive-compulsive disorders, and psychosis. This is in addition to psychiatric disorders like Tourette's Disorder, which are defined as repeated and objectively observable and measured behaviors (Eapen et al., 2019). Repetitive behaviors have also been identified as a major factor associated with certain types of dementia and neurocognitive disorders (Moheb et al., 2019).

Comparative psychopathology offers an avenue by which there can be new and more comprehensive ways of looking at psychological disorders and psychological constructs. We have shown in earlier chapters how the present status of studying psychopathology requires this sort of more comprehensive approach. There is also an argument to be made that the study of psychopathology could benefit by "going back to the drawing board" and looking objectively at how much different psychological disorders actually differ from each other. There certainly is a need to be specific if treatments will be effective. Still, there is also a case to be made that there is a benefit in recognizing similarities between conditions. This has potential benefit for mental health treatment as recognition of similarities could support a movement away from polypharmacy and the presence of so many different psychotherapy and counseling approaches. To determine whether there is a need as exists now for so many different treatments, suppose psychological disorders can be defined by symptoms with common etiologies similar across disorders, even if they have different elements (e.g., verbal vs. nonverbal). In that case, practitioners may find ways of emphasizing certain effective treatment methods for many different conditions. Targeting treatments in this way (e.g., allowing practitioners to focus on certain major psychological patterns) rather than trying to address a wide variety of different symptoms can only help benefit mental healthcare's effectiveness worldwide.

This chapter also addressed the possibility that a comprehensive approach like comparative psychopathology could benefit veterinary medicine. In many ways, veterinary psychiatry faces more difficulties than human psychiatry, as there does not seem to be any one method for defining psychopathology. Human psychiatry may suffer from having too many methods for understanding and treating psychiatric conditions, but veterinary medicine does not seem to have any. It is a recognized field of study that appears to lack any sort of formalized and structured approach. It is certainly not the case that the same method for understanding psychopathology in nonhuman animals has to be the same as that used for humans. It is also the case that a method of understanding and studying nonhuman animal psychopathology would require an approach noticeably different from one for human psychopathology given that verbal communication could not be emphasized (recall that verbal communication was one part of the RDoC method discussed earlier that has to be removed when studying nonhuman animals). However, having a method that incorporates a large part of the same approaches used for human and nonhuman animals could go a long way in providing direction for what seems presently to be a rather nondirectional approach to veterinary psychiatry. Comparative psychopathology as it stands now could help improve the study and treatment of human psychopathology while also helping advance direction to the study of nonhuman animal psychopathology.

References

Alhetheli, G., Alhammad, S., Almazyad, F., Algosair, I., Bukhari, A., Alayidi, S., & Almishali, F. (2022). Skin picking and trichotillomania disorders in the era of COVID-19: Cross-sectional study. *Journal of Pharmaceutical Negative Results*, 1930–1935.

Amodeo, D. A., Pahua, A. E., Zarate, M., Taylor, J. A., Peterson, S., Posadas, R. & Amodeo, L. (2019). Differences in the expression of restricted, repetitive behaviors in female and male BTBR T+ tf/J mice. *Behavioral Brain Research, 372,* 112028.

Aziziaram, S., & Basharpoor, S. (2020). The role of rumination, emotion regulation, and responsiveness to stress in predicting coronavirus (COVID-19) among nurses. *Quarterly Journal of Nursing Management, 9*(3), 8–18.

Bashaw, M. J., Gibson, M. D., Schowe, D. M., & Kucher, A. S. (2016). Does enrichment improve reptile welfare? Leopard geckos (Eublepharis macularius) respond to five types of environmental enrichment. *Applied Animal Behavior Science, 184,* 150–160.

Beck, A. T. (1991). Cognitive therapy: A 30-year retrospective. *American Psychologist, 46*(4), 368.

Bergström, I., Kilteni, K., & Slater, M. (2016). First-person perspective virtual body posture influences stress: A virtual reality body ownership study. *PLoS One, 11*(2), e0148060.

Cacioppo, J. T., Cacioppo, S., & Boomsma, D. I. (2014). Evolutionary mechanisms for loneliness. *Cognition & Emotion, 28*(1), 3–21.

Capitanio, J. P. (2018). Behavioral inhibition in nonhuman primates: The elephant in the room. *Behavioral Inhibition: Integrating Theory, Research, and Clinical Perspectives,* 17–33.

Caponnetto, P., Benenati, A., & Maglia, M. G. (2021). Psychopathological impact and resilient scenarios in inpatient with schizophrenia spectrum disorders related to Covid physical distancing policies: A systematic review. *Behavioral Sciences, 11*(4), 49.

Carroll, J. B. (1944). The analysis of verbal behavior. *Psychological Review, 51*(2), 102–119.

Chmielewski, M., Clark, L. A., Bagby, R. M., & Watson, D. (2015). Method matters: Understanding diagnostic reliability in *DSM-IV* and *DSM-5*. *Journal of Abnormal Psychology, 124*(3), 764–769. https://doi.org/10.1037/abn0000069

Cook, L., Mostazir, M., & Watkins, E. (2019). Reducing stress and preventing depression (RESPOND): Randomized controlled trial of web-based rumination-focused cognitive behavioral therapy for high-ruminating university students. *Journal of Medical Internet Research, 21*(5), e11349.

d'Angelo, D., Sacchettino, L., Carpentieri, R., Avallone, L., Gatta, C., & Napolitano, F. (2022). An interdisciplinary approach for compulsive behavior in dogs: a case report. *Frontiers in Veterinary Science, 9,* 801636.

Dahlen, A., Zarei, M., Melgoza, A., Wagle, M., & Guo, S. (2021). THC-induced behavioral stereotypy in zebrafish as a model of psychosis-like behavior. *Scientific Reports, 11*(1), 15693.

Dang, J., King, K. M., & Inzlicht, M. (2020). Why are self-report and behavioral measures weakly correlated? *Trends in Cognitive Sciences, 24*(4), 267–269.

Dereix-Calonge, I., Ruiz, F. J., Sierra, M. A., Pena-Vargas, A., & Ramírez, E. S. (2019). Acceptance and commitment training focused on repetitive negative thinking for clinical psychology trainees: A randomized controlled trial. *Journal of Contextual Behavioral Science, 12,* 81–88.

Dinwoodie, I. R., Dwyer, B., Zottola, V., Gleason, D., & Dodman, N. H. (2019). Demographics and comorbidity of behavior problems in dogs. *Journal of Veterinary Behavior, 32,* 62–71.

Dobson, H., & Smith, R. F. (2000). What is stress, and how does it affect reproduction?. *Animal Reproduction Science, 60,* 743–752.

Dos Santos, E. R. R., de Paula, J. L. S., Tardieux, F. M., Costa-e-Silva, V. N., Lal, A., & Leite, A. F. B. (2021). Association between COVID-19 and anxiety during social isolation: A systematic review. *World Journal of Clinical Cases*, *9*(25), 7433.

Eapen, V., McPherson, S., Karlov, L., Nicholls, L., Črnčec, R., & Mulligan, A. (2019). Social communication deficits and restricted repetitive behavior symptoms in Tourette syndrome. *Neuropsychiatric disease and treatment*, 2151–2160.

Ehring, T., & Watkins, E. R. (2008). Repetitive negative thinking as a transdiagnostic process. *International Journal of Cognitive Therapy*, *1*(3), 192–205.

Eissa, N., Azimullah, S., Jayaprakash, P., Jayaraj, R. L., Reiner, D., Ojha, S. K. & Sadek, B. (2019). The dual-active histamine H3 receptor antagonist and acetylcholine esterase inhibitor E100 ameliorates stereotyped repetitive behavior and neuroinflammmation in sodium valproate induced autism in mice. *Chemico-Biological Interactions*, *312*, 108775.

Eszlari, N., Millinghoffer, A., Petschner, P., Gonda, X., Baksa, D., Pulay, A. J. & Juhasz, G. (2019). Genome-wide association analysis reveals KCTD12 and miR-383-binding genes in the background of rumination. *Translational Psychiatry*, *9*(1), 119.

Epel, E. S., Crosswell, A. D., Mayer, S. E., Prather, A. A., Slavich, G. M., Puterman, E., & Mendes, W. B. (2018). More than a feeling: A unified view of stress measurement for population science. *Frontiers in Neuroendocrinology*, *49*, 146–169.

Eszlari, N., Bruncsics, B., Millinghoffer, A., Hullam, G., Petschner, P., Gonda, X. & Juhasz, G. (2021). Biology of perseverative negative thinking: the role of timing and folate intake. *Nutrients*, *13*(12), 4396.

Feldhaus, C. G., Jacobs, R. H., Watkins, E. R., Peters, A. T., Bessette, K. L., & Langenecker, S. A. (2020). Rumination-focused cognitive behavioral therapy decreases anxiety and increases behavioral activation among remitted adolescents. *Journal of Child and Family Studies*, *29*, 1982–1991.

Feng, X., & Wang, J. (2022). Presleep ruminating on intrusive thoughts increased the possibility of dreaming of threatening events. *Frontiers in Psychology*, *13*, 809131.

Fett, A. K. J., Hanssen, E., Eemers, M., Peters, E., & Shergill, S. S. (2022). Social isolation and psychosis: an investigation of social interactions and paranoia in daily life. *European Archives of Psychiatry and Clinical Neuroscience*, *272*(1), 119–127.

Ganellen, R. J. (2014). Assessing normal and abnormal personality functioning: Strengths and weaknesses of self-report, observer, and performance-based methods. *Personality Assessment in the DSM-5*, 17–27.

Garcia, J. & Gustavson, A.R. (1997). The science of self-report. In: *Observer* (January, 1997). Association of Psychological Science.

Gandhi, T., & Lee, C. C. (2021). Neural mechanisms underlying repetitive behaviors in rodent models of autism spectrum disorders. *Frontiers in Cellular Neuroscience*, *14*, 592710.

Goodwin, G. M. (2015). The overlap between anxiety, depression, and obsessive-compulsive disorder. *Dialogues in Clinical Neuroscience*, *17*(3), 249–260.

Goossens, L., Van Roekel, E., Verhagen, M., Cacioppo, J. T., Cacioppo, S., Maes, M., & Boomsma, D. I. (2015). The genetics of loneliness: Linking evolutionary theory to genome-wide genetics, epigenetics, and social science. *Perspectives on Psychological Science*, *10*(2), 213–226.

Grand, A. P., Kuhar, C. W., Leighty, K. A., Bettinger, T. L., & Laudenslager, M. L. (2012). Using personality ratings and cortisol to characterize individual differences in African Elephants (Loxodonta africana). *Applied Animal Behaviour Science*, *142*(1–2), 69–75.

Haller, H., Breilmann, P., Schröter, M., Dobos, G., & Cramer, H. (2021). A systematic review and meta-analysis of acceptance-and mindfulness-based interventions for DSM-5 anxiety disorders. *Scientific Reports, 11*(1), 20385.

Hale, L., & Hale, B. (2010). Treat the source not the symptoms: why thinking about sleep informs the social determinants of health. *Health Education Research, 25*(3), 395–400.

Harlow, H. F., & Harlow, M. K. (1962). The effect of rearing conditions on behavior. *Bulletin of the Menninger Clinic, 26*(5), 213.

Harlow, H. F., & Suomi, S. J. (1971). Production of depressive behaviors in young monkeys. *Journal of Autism and Childhood Schizophrenia, 1*(3), 246–255.

Hasegawa, A., Oura, S. I., Yamamoto, T., Kunisato, Y., Matsuda, Y., & Adachi, M. (2023). Causes and consequences of stress generation: Longitudinal associations of negative events, aggressive behaviors, rumination, and depressive symptoms. *Current Psychology, 42*(18), 15708–15717.

Heatley Tejada, A., Dunbar, R. I. M., & Montero, M. (2020). Physical contact and loneliness: being touched reduces perceptions of loneliness. *Adaptive Human Behavior and Physiology, 6*, 292–306.

Helle, A. C., Trull, T. J., Watts, A. L., McDowell, Y., & Sher, K. J. (2020). Psychiatric comorbidity as a function of severity: DSM-5 alcohol use disorder and HiTOP classification of mental disorders. *Alcoholism: Clinical and Experimental Research, 44*(3), 632–644.

Horne, P. J., & Lowe, C. F. (1997). Toward a theory of verbal behavior. *Journal of the Experimental Analysis of Behavior, 68*(2), 271–296.

Horie, K., Inoue, K., Suzuki, S., Adachi, S., Yada, S., Hirayama, T. & Nishimori, K. (2019). Oxytocin receptor knockout prairie voles generated by CRISPR/Cas9 editing show reduced preference for social novelty and exaggerated repetitive behaviors. *Hormones and Behavior, 111*, 60–69.

Jacob, Y., Morris, L. S., Huang, K. H., Schneider, M., Rutter, S., Verma, G. & Balchandani, P. (2020). Neural correlates of rumination in major depressive disorder: A brain network analysis. *NeuroImage: Clinical, 25*, 102142.

Katz, M., Corson, F., Keil, W., Singhal, A., Bae, A., Lu, Y. & Shaham, S. (2019). Glutamate spillover in C. elegans triggers repetitive behavior through presynaptic activation of MGL-2/mGluR5. *Nature Communications, 10*(1), 1882.

Keefer, K. V. (2015). Self-report assessments of emotional competencies: A critical look at methods and meanings. *Journal of Psychoeducational Assessment, 33*(1), 3–23. https://doi.org/10.1177/0734282914550381

Kirk, R. G., & Ramsden, E. (2018). Working across species down on the farm: Howard S. Liddell and the development of comparative psychopathology, c. 1923–1962. *History and Philosophy of the Life Sciences, 40*, 1–29.

Keller, F. M., Derksen, C., Kötting, L., Dahmen, A., & Lippke, S. (2023). Distress, loneliness, and mental health during the COVID-19 pandemic: Test of the extension of the Evolutionary Theory of Loneliness. *Applied Psychology: Health and Well-Being, 15*(1), 24–48.

Kelly, A. D., & Kelly, M. E. (2022). Acceptance and commitment training in applied behavior analysis: where have you been all my life?. *Behavior Analysis in Practice, 15*(1), 43–54.

Kelly, E., Meng, F., Fujita, H., Morgado, F., Kazemi, Y., Rice, L. C. & Tsai, P. T. (2020). Regulation of autism-relevant behaviors by cerebellar–prefrontal cortical circuits. *Nature Neuroscience, 23*(9), 1102–1110.

Kogan, L. R., & Grigg, E. K. (2021). Laser light pointers for use in companion cat play: Association with guardian-reported abnormal repetitive behaviors. *Animals, 11*(8), 2178.

Koolhaas, J. M., De Boer, S. F., Buwalda, B., & Meerlo, P. (2017). Social stress models in rodents: Towards enhanced validity. *Neurobiology of Stress*, *6*, 104–112.

Kracker Imthon, A., Antônio Caldart, C., Do Rosário, M. C., Fontenelle, L. F., Constantino Miguel, E., & Arzeno Ferrão, Y. (2020). Stressful life events and the clinical expression of Obsessive–Compulsive Disorder (OCD): an exploratory study. *Journal of Clinical Medicine*, *9*(10), 3371.

Kukreja, S., Kalra, G., Shah, N., & Shrivastava, A. (2023). Polypharmacy in psychiatry: A review. *Mens Sana Monographs*, *11*(1), 82.

LaFrance, D. L., & Tarbox, J. (2020). The importance of multiple exemplar instruction in the establishment of novel verbal behavior. *Journal of Applied Behavior Analysis*, *53*(1), 10–24.

Langen, M., Durston, S., Kas, M. J., Van Engeland, H., & Staal, W. G. (2011a). The neurobiology of repetitive behavior:... and men. *Neuroscience & Biobehavioral Reviews*, *35*(3), 356–365.

Langen, M., Kas, M. J., Staal, W. G., van Engeland, H., & Durston, S. (2011b). The neurobiology of repetitive behavior: of mice.... *Neuroscience & Biobehavioral Reviews*, *35*(3), 345–355.

Lawrence, A. B., & Terlouw, E. C. (1993). A review of behavioral factors involved in the development and continued performance of stereotypic behaviors in pigs. *Journal of Animal Science*, *71*(10), 2815–2825.

Levine, S. (1985). A definition of stress?. In: *Animal Stress* (pp. 51–69). New York, NY: Springer New York.

Lewis, M. H., Tanimura, Y., Lee, L. W., & Bodfish, J. W. (2007). Animal models of restricted repetitive behavior in autism. *Behavioural Brain Research*, *176*(1), 66–74.

Luiselli, J. K. (2015). Behavioral treatment of rumination: Research and clinical applications. *Journal of Applied Behavior Analysis*, *48*(3), 707–711.

Lustberg, D., Iannitelli, A. F., Tillage, R. P., Pruitt, M., Liles, L. C., & Weinshenker, D. (2020). Central norepinephrine transmission is required for stress-induced repetitive behavior in two rodent models of obsessive-compulsive disorder. *Psychopharmacology*, *237*, 1973–1987.

Lustberg, D. J., Liu, J. Q., Iannitelli, A. F., Vanderhoof, S. O., Liles, L. C., McCann, K. E., & Weinshenker, D. (2022). Norepinephrine and dopamine contribute to distinct repetitive behaviors induced by novel odorant stress in male and female mice. *Hormones and Behavior*, *144*, 105205.

Mansueto, G., Cavallo, C., Palmieri, S., Ruggiero, G. M., Sassaroli, S., & Caselli, G. (2021). Adverse childhood experiences and repetitive negative thinking in adulthood: A systematic review. *Clinical Psychology & Psychotherapy*, *28*(3), 557–568.

Maple, T. L. (2007). Toward a science of welfare for animals in the zoo. *Journal of Applied Animal Welfare Science*, *10*(1), 63–70.

Martínez-González, A. E., Cervin, M., & Piqueras, J. A. (2022). Relationships between emotion regulation, social communication and repetitive behaviors in Autism Spectrum Disorder. *Journal of Autism and Developmental Disorders*, *52*(10), 4519–4527.

McCarty, R. (2020). Evolution of the stress concept. In: *Stress and Mental Disorders: Insights from Animal Models* (pp. 56–83). Oxford University Press.

McGuigan, F. J. (1970). Covert oral behavior during the silent performance of language tasks. *Psychological Bulletin*, *74*(5), 309–326. https://doi.org/10.1037/h0030082

Mezo, P. G., & Baker, R. M. (2012). The moderating effects of stress and rumination on depressive symptoms in women and men. *Stress and Health*, *28*(4), 333–339.

Migan-Gandonou, J. A., & Leon, Y. (2020). Empirically derived consequences to treat rumination. *Behavioral Interventions*, *35*(1), 166–177.

Mills, D. S., Demontigny-Bédard, I., Gruen, M., Klinck, M. P., McPeake, K. J., Barcelos, A. M. & Levine, E. (2020). Pain and problem behavior in cats and dogs. *Animals*, *10*(2), 318.

Moheb, N., Charuworn, K., Ashla, M. M., Desarzant, R., Chavez, D., & Mendez, M. F. (2019). Repetitive behaviors in frontotemporal dementia: Compulsions or impulsions?. *The Journal of Neuropsychiatry and Clinical Neurosciences*, *31*(2), 132–136.

Monteregge, S., Tsagkalidou, A., Cuijpers, P., & Spinhoven, P. (2020). The effects of different types of treatment for anxiety on repetitive negative thinking: A meta-analysis. *Clinical Psychology: Science and Practice*, *27*(2), e12316.

Mursaleen, M. (2023). Efficacy of online cognitive behavioral therapy for social anxiety disorder comorbid with depression. *Journal of Positive School Psychology*, *7*(6), 981–1007.

Nadeem, A., Ahmad, S. F., Al-Harbi, N. O., Attia, S. M., Alshammari, M. A., Alzahrani, K. S., & Bakheet, S. A. (2019). Increased oxidative stress in the cerebellum and peripheral immune cells leads to exaggerated autism-like repetitive behavior due to deficiency of antioxidant response in BTBR T+ tf/J mice. *Progress in Neuro-Psychopharmacology and Biological Psychiatry*, *89*, 245–253.

Nuttgens, S. (2023). Of interventive doppelgangers and other barriers to evidence-based practice in psychotherapy. *Journal of Psychotherapy Integration*, *33*(1), 20.

Oliveirra, E. C. B., Fitzpatrick, C. L., Kim, H. S., Gulassa, D. C. R., Amaral, R. S., de Mattos Cristiana, N. & Tavares, H. (2019). Obsessive–compulsive or addiction? Categorical diagnostic analysis of excoriation disorder compared to obsessive-compulsive disorder and gambling disorder. *Psychiatry Research*, *281*, 112518.

Perez Garcia, G., Perez, G. M., De Gasperi, R., Gama Sosa, M. A., Otero-Pagan, A., Pryor, D. & Elder, G. A. (2021). Progressive cognitive and post-traumatic stress disorder-related behavioral traits in rats exposed to repetitive low-level blast. *Journal of Neurotrauma*, *38*(14), 2030–2045.

Puta, C., Steidten, T., Baumbach, P., Wöhrl, T., May, R., Kellmann, M., ... & Gabriel, H. H. (2018). Standardized assessment of resistance training-induced subjective symptoms and objective signs of immunological stress responses in young athletes. *Frontiers in Physiology*, *9*, 698.

Reichert, R. A., Martins, G. D. G., da Silva, A. M. B., Scatena, A., Barbugli, B. C., De Micheli, D., & Andrade, A. L. M. (2021). New forms of addiction: digital media. *Psychology of substance abuse: Psychotherapy, clinical management and social intervention*, 43–53.

Rice, S., Seidler, Z., Kealy, D., Ogrodniczuk, J., Zajac, I., & Oliffe, J. (2022). Men's depression, externalizing, and DSM-5-TR: primary signs and symptoms or co-occurring symptoms?. *Harvard Review of Psychiatry*, *30*(5), 317–322.

Ruiz, F. J., Flórez, C. L., García-Martín, M. B., Monroy-Cifuentes, A., Barreto-Montero, K., García-Beltrán, D. M. & Gil-Luciano, B. (2018). A multiple-baseline evaluation of a brief acceptance and commitment therapy protocol focused on repetitive negative thinking for moderate emotional disorders. *Journal of Contextual Behavioral Science*, *9*, 1–14.

Schouten, W., Rushen, J., & De Passillé, A. M. B. (1991). Stereotypic behavior and heart rate in pigs. *Physiology & Behavior*, *50*(3), 617–624.

Santore, L. A., Gerber, A., Gioia, A. N., Bianchi, R., Talledo, F., Peris, T. S., & Lerner, M. D. (2020). Felt but not seen: Observed restricted repetitive behaviors are associated with self-report—but not parent-report—obsessive-compulsive disorder symptoms in youth with autism spectrum disorder. *Autism*, *24*(4), 983–994.

Spinhoven, P., Klein, N., Kennis, M., Cramer, A. O., Siegle, G., Cuijpers, P. & Bockting, C. L. (2018). The effects of cognitive-behavior therapy for depression on repetitive negative thinking: A meta-analysis. *Behaviour Research and Therapy*, *106*, 71–85.

Spithoven, A. W., Cacioppo, S., Goossens, L., & Cacioppo, J. T. (2019). Genetic contributions to loneliness and their relevance to the evolutionary theory of loneliness. *Perspectives on Psychological Science*, *14*(3), 376–396.

Stott, G. H. (1981). What is animal stress and how is it measured?. *Journal of Animal Science*, *52*(1), 150–153.

Sulkama, S., Salonen, M., Mikkola, S., Hakanen, E., Puurunen, J., Araujo, C. & Hanne, L. (2022). Aggressiveness, ADHD-like behaviour, and environment influence repetitive behaviour in dogs. *Science Reports*, *12*, 3520. https://doi.org/10.1038/s41598-022-07443-6

Suomi, S. J., Harlow, H. F., & Domek, C. J. (1970). Effect of repetitive infant-infant separation of young monkeys. *Journal of Abnormal Psychology*, *76*(2), 161.

Szejko, N., & Müller-Vahl, K. R. (2021). Challenges in the diagnosis and assessment in patients with Tourette syndrome and comorbid obsessive-compulsive disorder. *Neuropsychiatric Disease and Treatment*, 1253–1266.

Taborsky, M. (2014). Tribute to Tinbergen: the four problems of biology. A critical appraisal. *Ethology*, *120*(3), 224–227.

Tackman, A. M., Sbarra, D. A., Carey, A. L., Donnellan, M. B., Horn, A. B., Holtzman, N. S. & Mehl, M. R. (2019). Depression, negative emotionality, and self-referential language: A multi-lab, multi-measure, and multi-language-task research synthesis. *Journal of Personality and Social Psychology*, *116*(5), 817.

Taylor, M. M., & Snyder, H. R. (2021). Repetitive negative thinking shared across rumination and worry predicts symptoms of depression and anxiety. *Journal of Psychopathology and Behavioral Assessment*, *43*(4), 904–915.

Tichenor, S. E., & Yaruss, J. S. (2021). Variability of stuttering: Behavior and impact. *American Journal of Speech-Language Pathology*, *30*(1), 75–88.

Tonna, M., Ponzi, D., Palanza, P., Marchesi, C., & Parmigiani, S. (2020). Proximate and ultimate causes of ritual behavior. *Behavioural Brain Research*, *393*, 112772.

Watkins, E. R. (2018). *Rumination-focused cognitive-behavioral therapy for depression*. Guilford Publications.

Watkins, E. R., & Roberts, H. (2020). Reflecting on rumination: Consequences, causes, mechanisms and treatment of rumination. *Behaviour Research and Therapy*, *127*, 103573.

Wiggins, L. D., Rice, C. E., Barger, B., Soke, G. N., Lee, L. C., Moody, E. & Levy, S. E. (2019). DSM-5 criteria for autism spectrum disorder maximizes diagnostic sensitivity and specificity in preschool children. *Social Psychiatry and Psychiatric Epidemiology*, *54*, 693–701.

Wilkialis, L., Rodrigues, N. B., Cha, D. S., Siegel, A., Majeed, A., Lui, L. M. & McIntyre, R. S. (2021). Social isolation, loneliness and generalized anxiety: implications and associations during the COVID-19 quarantine. *Brain Sciences*, *11*(12), 1620.

Williams, K. L., Campi, E., & Baranek, G. T. (2021). Associations among sensory hyperresponsiveness, restricted and repetitive behaviors, and anxiety in autism: An integrated systematic review. *Research in Autism Spectrum Disorders*, *83*, 101763.

Woods, K. E., Luiselli, J. K., & Tomassone, S. (2013). Functional analysis and intervention for chronic rumination. *Journal of Applied Behavior Analysis*, *46*(1), 328–332.

Yamada, R., Kuze-Arata, S., Kiyokawa, Y., & Takeuchi, Y. (2019). Prevalence of 25 canine behavioral problems and relevant factors of each behavior in Japan. *Journal of Veterinary Medical Science, 81*(8), 1090–1096.

Yoo, T., Kim, S. G., Yang, S. H., Kim, H., Kim, E., & Kim, S. Y. (2020). A DLG2 deficiency in mice leads to reduced sociability and increased repetitive behavior accompanied by aberrant synaptic transmission in the dorsal striatum. *Molecular Autism, 11*(1), 1–14.

Zagaria, A., Ballesio, A., Vacca, M., & Lombardo, C. (2023). Repetitive negative thinking as a central node between psychopathological domains: A network analysis. *International Journal of Cognitive Therapy, 16*(2), 143–160.

Zhang, H., Sollmann, N., Castrillón, G., Kurcyus, K., Meyer, B., Zimmer, C., & Krieg, S. M. (2020). Intranetwork and internetwork effects of navigated transcranial magnetic stimulation using low-and high-frequency pulse application to the dorsolateral prefrontal cortex: a combined rTMS–fMRI approach. *Journal of Clinical Neurophysiology, 37*(2), 131–139.

Zimmerman, M., Kerr, S., Kiefer, R., Balling, C., & Dalrymple, K. (2019). What is anxious depression? Overlap and agreement between different definitions. *Journal of Psychiatric Research, 109*, 133–138.

Zorzo, C., Méndez-López, M., Méndez, M., & Arias, J. L. (2019). Adult social isolation leads to anxiety and spatial memory impairment: Brain activity pattern of COx and c-Fos. *Behavioural Brain Research, 365*, 170–177.

6 Comparative Psychopathology and Dementia

Introduction

Within the past several decades, psychologists and other nonmedical professionals have become more involved in understanding and treating age-related psychological conditions. This previously was the domain primarily of psychiatrists and neurologists, but the emphasis has been on understanding these conditions from a behavioral perspective rather than a medical one. When it comes to considering psychological disorders associated with aging, Alzheimer's Disease is the most common type, but there are others. "Dementia" is the medical term for the change in brain functioning associated with physiological changes, and "Major Neurocognitive Disorder" is the psychological term for the cognitive deficits associated with those medical conditions. Changes in memory, attention, and comprehension are three main areas often impacted by dementia.

Although dementia is a medical condition, its drastic negative impact is largely a social one. Dementia leaves its victims unable to communicate effectively with others around them. This is devastating to families as elderly relatives succumb to dementia's effects and forget not only who they are but also how to communicate with other people. Making this even more devastating is that the victims of dementia also fail how to effectively interact with all aspects of their social environment and even get to the point where they can no longer do things necessary for survival. It is an unfortunate aspect of Alzheimer's Disease that one of the main ways it is terminal is that individuals with Alzheimer's Disease forget things to the point that they forget how to swallow and breathe.

It is devastating for family members to watch someone they care about suffer the impact of dementia. They see the person having less and less ability to remember things and function in the social world. Making the effects of dementia even more upsetting are behavioral problems associated with this disorder. Families watch loved ones forget important things and become verbally agitated frequently. Individuals with dementia often engage in

DOI: 10.4324/9781003408918-7

agitated and disruptive behaviors that seem directly related to their confusion and difficulties in understanding and interacting with the social world. Caretakers of individuals with dementia seek help but may find it difficult because the causes of these agitated and disruptive behaviors can be so difficult to understand.

Recognizing what makes understanding agitated behaviors in dementia so challenging requires some specifics about the behaviors and how they differ from what would often be expected. They present difficulties because the person with dementia simply is not acting in ways that make sense given what we humans expect of other humans expressing emotional distress. Individuals with dementia often yell and scream about needing help but will not show a decrease in their distress level, even if someone tries to help them. An example would be someone with dementia yelling out "Help Me!!" but continuing to yell this even when someone comes to try and help them. Having help from someone, the apparent goal of what the individual was yelling, does not help lessen the emotional distress triggering the behavior. When someone asks for help, getting help is usually expected to reduce the person's emotional distress. Having this not happen can cause considerable concern for caregivers trying to help someone with dementia.

Memory problems also complicate the difficulties associated with dementia. When an older adult with dementia yells out for help because they need to care for young children, even when everyone knows that the person's children are adults living on their own, it is challenging to figure out how to help lessen the person's distress. That situation becomes even more complicated when attempts to address the person's confused concerns do not help. One example many caregivers of people with dementia face is a confused individual who insists that someone call their spouse to let them know that they will not be home and that the spouse needs to watch the young children. A common and sensible response to this might be to pick up the phone, pretend to call the spouse, and say that the person will not be home and they should watch the children. Even though this might be seen as a lie, pretending to call someone who is not actually on the other line, many people will think this lie acceptable if it helps the person not worry so much. This type of situation tends to be difficult because the approach often does not work. The approach of pretending to call the person's spouse about the young children usually does not lessen the person's distress and agitated behaviors. The confused individual will often continue the yelling and distressed behaviors even after being told that the spouse was called.

What all this shows is that understanding and addressing agitated behaviors in someone with dementia is complicated and does not follow the social rules humans often associate with agitated behaviors. We often look at yelling about needing help as a behavior that occurs to try and get other people to do something specific to address a particular problem. Yelling is a form of verbal communication, as the typical expectation goes, pointing to one specific needed response in a way that clarifies that the response must be done urgently. Raising the volume of what is said is a way of emphasizing the importance and urgency of what precisely is being said.

Looking at difficulties associated with agitated behaviors in dementia shows that they do not follow the rules expected of yelling in typical human social environments. Words do not have the same meaning (i.e., pointing to something specific that needs to be done), and the yelling seems to have even more importance than it might otherwise be. Yelling and repetitiveness appear more significant than specifically what is being said. How the confused distress is expressed has primacy over what words or nonverbal gestures are used.

Agitated behaviors have been identified as one of the most distressing aspects of dementia caregiving. It leads not only to stress for the person who has dementia but also for the caregiver. Petrovsky et al. (2020) interviewed 250 caregivers of dementia patients and found that over half saw their harsh communication increase towards the patients due to stress caused by agitated behaviors. Words that have very little connection to what is happening, such as what occurs with agitated verbal behaviors in dementia, elicit words from caregivers that are more emotional than functional. All of these lead to situations where anger is more and more prevalent in behaviors, and very little of it effectively decreases emotional distress. This would reflect one important reason for trying to gain a better sense of what the agitated behaviors are signaling.

Agitated behaviors often arise because of unmet needs (Minyo & Judge, 2020). Individuals with mild to moderate dementia are often able to express their unmet needs when interviewed and constantly have agitated behaviors like yelling coinciding with these unmet needs. Agitated behaviors, in this way, serve as the primary way that someone with dementia expresses that something is wrong. What the person is trying to accomplish with the yelling changes based on the emotional characteristics of the situation. This includes what situations the person finds themselves in, how other people are responding, and what resources the person has readily available. The frequency and severity of agitated behaviors changed depending on the structure of nursing homes (Testad et al., 2010).

Verbal language is the primary way that humans express cognitive processes. Humans get concerned about something needing to be done and point it out using words. If the person has interpreted cognitively that the situation needs to be addressed urgently, then yelling is used. This raised voice is often seen as a way of emphasizing what is being said. Humans often consider the words to have primacy rather than the yelling itself. This makes more sense when the person can accurately use words to express what they are experiencing cognitively. Dementia takes away the accuracy of words, and identifying what the person with dementia needs requires a decreased emphasis on words. It requires looking at the aspects of yelling and agitation as forms of vocalization, separate from the words used as part of those behaviors.

Vocalizations emphasizing the "how" distress is being expressed, rather than the "what" in terms of what specifically needs to be addressed, are common in the nonhuman animal social world. Nonhuman animals do not use words, so the focus on vocalizations is not on specifics as much as with humans. Noises are used to gain social support and alert others to dangers without eliciting a specific behavioral response. Vocalizations are used to gather assistance and make others aware rather than trying to get them to exert some sort of defined response.

Animals use vocalizations to get attention and gather support from others. Words are not used and are unnecessary since the purpose is not to point out anything specific. As pointed out in previous chapters, animals treat each situation as a unique experience, so there is no need to show any relationship to previous experiences. Animals may rely on previous learning for responses but do not rely on a need for shared experiences to get others to respond similarly to shared past experiences. There is a need to get support from others, but not having shared experiences forms the basis for responding.

This chapter will consider the possibility that humans suffering from dementia may be responding to distress situations similar to how nonhumans respond. By having less ability to use verbal speech effectively, there may be a reliance on yelling and behaviors others might call "agitated" to respond to emotional distress. Much like nonhuman animals, humans with dementia may use vocalizations to gain support and trigger awareness of perceived dangers rather than trying to get any specific outcome. Achieving a feeling of community and support may be the goal rather than getting other people to say something or do something geared to a clear outcome. What the person with dementia may be looking for is that feeling of support and a clear sense that their warnings have been heeded. That may take considerable time and effort, but it is not likely to be reached using words or attempts at specific behaviors to help address distressed concerns.

Comparing the purpose of vocalizations and changes in vocalization across species is not new and has been described as a "powerful tool" for understanding the purposes of vocalizations (Ravignani et al., 2019). In his book, *The Expression of Emotion in Man and Animals*, Charles Darwin (1872) postulated that vocalizations primarily express emotions rather than specific information. Providing specific information and/or directions is the primary function of words but not of vocalizations. Changes in tonality, beat, timescales, and temporal structures across species reflect complex social and behavioral processes (Kello et al., 2017). Vocalizations across animal species are used more to express emotions than to provide specific informa- tion and/or guidance (Maskeliunas et al., 2018; Scheumann et al., 2017). All of this shows reason to expect that yelling in dementia can effectively be explored as a type of vocalization meant to express emotion and gather social support rather than provide specific instructions or information.

Dog barking is one of the most researched types of vocalizations used by nonhuman animals. Like all nonhuman animals, dogs live in a social world that does not rely on words but different types of sounds for communica- tion. Much like humans with dementia, dogs cannot rely on their vocaliza- tions to carry specific information or to consistently relay information about how a present situation is similar to previous cases. Humans often use words to point out specific concerns and to connect with other people about how a present situation relates to others. But humans with dementia cannot rely on that ability, and dogs depending on barking for communication never rely on that ability. So, humans with dementia and agitated behaviors and dogs with barking are trying to navigate similar social milieus.

Below are two examples demonstrating similarities between the experi- ences of humans with dementia and nonhumans:

1. Mabel was a resident of a nursing home who had been diagnosed with Alzheimer's disease. She would frequently go up and down the hallway of her unit, yelling at people. She would yell about needing to leave to get home and make dinner for her husband and children. Staff at the nursing home were aware that her children were all grown and living on their own and that her husband had passed away several years ago. For these rea- sons, it was unclear why she was demanding to leave so that she could take care of them even though staff at the nursing home continued to remind her that she lived at the home and that her children were OK on their own. It was unclear to staff why she was engaging in this behavior. Making the behavior even more unclear were concerns about why she would continue to yell about needing to go home even after her behaviors were addressed by staff. When they provided supportive interventions that were meant to try and help her feel less distressed, this only seemed to serve as a means of making her more distressed. She would yell even louder and more frequently when staff would explain to her what was happening in terms of her being in the nursing home and not being in any danger. Even when the staff assured her that they would call her husband to tell him why she was late, Mabel continued to yell without showing any recognition that someone had just tried to address the very thing that upset her.

2. Roxy was a dog whom the same family had owned for seven years. She was generally healthy and would spend much time moving about the fam- ily's home. She would go up and down the hall and bark loudly whenever

there were any changes in the household. Her barking would continue multiple times and stop only when Roxy seemed to be waiting to determine if something still needed to be addressed. Even attempts to calm her down by her owners would usually not stop the barking. Interestingly, if other dogs were barking in the neighborhood when Roxy barked, their combined barking would continue until one of them stopped. At that point, all of them would stop, but it was clear that Roxy was waiting to see if there were any reasons to start barking again.

These two situations are considerably more similar than might seem to be the case initially. They both involve situations where an individual is trying to get across that something is bothering them. They also include situations where an individual continues to express concern even when it seems to others that the situation has been addressed. What is happening in both situations is that there is concern being expressed and that the concern is not necessarily something evident to others. Both concerns are somewhat generalized. Even when something specific is done to address the situation, it does not appear to decrease the level of emotional distress the person is exhibiting.

When human beings use words, there is a specificity to the process. People say something, and what they say points to an object or situation. Even if there are multiple aspects to the situation being referenced, the words are usually expected to refer to something specific. When we say something, it will reference something in the outside world. Not only is there an expectation that something is being referenced outside of the individual, but that there is a shared experience in terms of what the person addresses can also be seen and experienced by someone else.

Words are a type of verbalization used by humans. Other animals also have verbalizations but do not use them like humans use words. Verbalizations are used to call others' attention to something being wrong. They may be used as a "siren" warning that something is wrong but not necessarily specifying what is wrong. Even if the "siren" seems to be pointing towards something specific, it is not always the case that pointing this out is why the "siren" is being activated. Finding out what is wrong is considered more of a communal responsibility. One individual points out that something is wrong, and then it is up to the group to determine the specifics and address the situation. There is a role each individual has in letting someone know something is wrong, and then it is more of a social responsibility to fix the situation.

Barking is this sort of "siren." Dogs bark as a way of letting others know that they perceive a problem in their immediate vicinity. It may be that the dog points towards the specific problem when barking, but in many ways, this is more coincidental than it is direction. They are not barking to necessarily point out where the problem is but that a problem exists. This is a warning to others and is also a call for assistance. It may be that the dog does know what needs to be addressed, but that is not the main reason for barking. Dogs usually bark to let people know that a problem exists to avoid the situation or to get assistance in trying to address what is happening. Barking is used to bring other individuals into the situation so that there is more of a group understanding of what is happening and a social connection in facing the problem.

What barking shows is that dogs communicate to try to bring other people into the social scenario. They are barking to get others into the situation for help or acknowledgment. If it is an attempt for acknowledgement, this ensures that people recognize what is happening. Dogs are not trying to say, "There is a problem over there that I am going to fix," but instead are trying to say, "There is a problem around us, and we either need to fix it together or others need to avoid this situation." That is why trying to fix a situation may not necessarily stop the barking. If a human goes over to a barking dog, perceives that they know the problem, and then tries to fix it, the dog may still perceive that a problem exists and continue to experience a sense that "I need to let other individuals know what is happening."

Understanding barking in this way led Yin and McCowan to describe dog barking as an "...attention-seeking vocalization rather than a context-specific form of communication." (Yin & McCowan, 2004). Notice here that the focus is on getting others to pay attention to what is happening. Barking is a method for obtaining the attention that something is problematic and/or potentially dangerous. These barks are often used to get others to focus on something else that is going on. This could include noises like doorbells, the approach of a potentially hostile other dog, or isolation. Barking also occurs with play, which could reflect how affective changes contribute to barking. Something leads the dog to feel different, and alerting to the presence of this change is why barking occurs.

Barking is a social behavior similar to those exhibited by other animals. This includes scream vocalizations from certain types of macaques. These social behaviors are used to recruit support from allies against opponents (Gouzoules & Gouzoules, 1989) and occur with other animals, like recess monkeys. Vocalizations are used as a way of getting other individuals to provide help in dangerous situations. It is not always clear what specific type of danger is being experienced, but what is clear is the social aspect of trying to get other people involved. It may be that the vocalizations are used in specific contexts, but not that the attempt is to get anything specific done. What is more important is getting allies to help in fighting off whatever danger there is. Still, at the moment, the vocalizations are not meant to focus the individuals on any one particular type of danger or problem.

Barking is often used to try to regain a social group, which could explain why dogs who bark may only bark louder when someone yells at them to stop barking. Dogs often respond to someone yelling at them with more barking because they may interpret the yelling as the individual essentially barking back at them (McGreevy, 2004). Barking is a behavior by which dogs express emotional states. It does not appear to be a way that dogs communicate directly with other dogs. Barking serves as a way of announcing that something is wrong and emotionally distressing but is not necessarily geared towards getting something specific to happen (Pongracz et al., 2010). In this way, it differs considerably from what humans expect from verbal speech. Dogs have very distinct barks and can be identified based on different aspects of their barks (Perez-Espinosa et al., 2018).

When discussing another purpose of barking, Ruusila and Pesonen (2004) discussed how hunters can be more successful in finding and hunting moose if a dog is with them. In these situations, the dog will bark at the moose to halter it, and the hunter can approach the moose to get into the shooting range. This can be more successful if a dog is barking at the moose. Notice how, in this situation, it is not the case that the dog is telling the hunter to kill the moose. There is no specific relationship where the dog points at the moose to get a specific action directed toward a specific target. Hunting success is increased when a dog is available to help with the hunt. But it is not the case that the dog is necessarily involved with the hunter in terms of planning on the moose being shot and killed. Moreover, there is cooperation between the hunter and the dog regarding recognizing that the moose needs to be stopped. The dog is barking at the moose to get some control over a huge animal, which could cause some problems for the group.

Dogs in large social groups where moose hunting is necessary are taught to track the moose and bring it into the hunter's shooting range. But it is not the case that the dog is necessarily telling the hunter to shoot the moose. The training involves getting the dog to recognize that a moose is in the area and that it needs to be directed to a particular place so that something can be done. There is no indication that the dog is telling the hunter to do something specific like shoot the moose but more that the dog is generally directing the moose in a way that it has been trained to do and is barking as a way of getting the situation to turn out in a certain general way. A situation needs to be addressed, and the dog is doing its part to announce what needs to be done.

Some researchers have suggested that barking is essentially nonfunctional (Yin, 2002) beyond having the purpose of developing a sense of social connectedness. Authors addressing the social importance of barking show that types of social interactions strongly influence vocalizations like barking. There is a considerable difference between the types of barking in terms of context, and this suggests that the social environment plays a role in determining what sorts of barks are used. They were barking in different ways, bringing about a sense that others were involved and concerned about what was happening. Dogs use different types of barking to announce different things to the social group and even differ in barking based on whether the targeted response is from other dogs or humans.

Barking during separation is an example showing that its purpose often brings about a sense of connectedness when facing stressful situations. When dealing with separation, younger dogs bark more than older dogs. This is attributed to younger dogs being more excitable and more prone to experiencing stress earlier than older dogs (Pongracz et al., 2017). When dogs see separation from their owner as stressful, this tends to lead them to bark louder and more often. This issue tends to occur more with younger dogs than older dogs. This research indicates the degree to which barking is often related to stress and not necessarily related to any specific goal. It is a way of decreasing the degree to which the individual dog is experiencing stress about the owner being away or otherwise being separated from the owner.

What is interesting to consider with all this is the degree to which barking in dogs and yelling in individuals with dementia have similar purposes. They are both ways of expressing stress and trying to gain some control over the situation causing the stress. Neither behavior seems to have any specific goal other than trying to express feelings of stress and get social support from others. That assistance may not be anything specific other than getting some sense of social support. This social aspect is particularly interesting as both barking and yelling are ways of gaining support and assistance from others. It is not necessarily the case that barking has any specific goal related directly to the behavior other than trying to alert others that there is a problem and that assistance is needed. In this way, it is much like yelling in dementia, where there is a degree to which the person is trying to express difficulties and get assistance in that situation. Neither of these behaviors seemed geared towards getting any specific assistance but rather to get a sense that other people are hearing the alarm and heeding the call for assistance.

Different dog barks relay different types of emotional material (Jegh-Czinege et al., 2020). Dogs react differently to the different barks of other dogs. Those reactions can be barking back or other types of verbalizations. If dogs are close, it may also take the form of getting closer to each other. What is interesting to note here is that what the barking does not typically elicit are dogs doing something specific to fix a problem. If dogs are brought to an area where they see something that needs response, this situation may elicit some behavior. However, the barking brings the dogs to the area as a way of gathering in response to a situation rather than directing specific behaviors geared toward fixing it.

Vocalizations like barking seek to develop a sense of community support around a problem. Dogs want to bring others together to feel supported in what they face. Agitated verbal behaviors from individuals with dementia may be geared to elicit the same response. These behaviors look to elicit support and a sense of community involvement from others around the person with dementia. Even if the words are used, they are not geared to elicit any specific response or behavior from others. It is more a search to gather others around to lessen feelings of emotional distress rather than to get something done to fix the situation causing the distress.

It is interesting to consider that the view of dementia reflected in this chapter forms the central thesis of "validation therapy" (Fell, 2014). In this approach to therapy with dementia, the "validation worker" recognizes that words are ineffective for the individual in addressing immediate needs. Individuals with dementia are looking to find safety, comfort, and emotional support in environments where they feel estranged from other people. Validation therapy focuses on supporting the emotional content of the individuals' words and behaviors. These vocalizations express a need for connectedness, support, and safety from others, and the "validation worker" works on addressing the emotional content behind the individual's behaviors.

Other therapeutic interventions for dementia also show that using words is of minimal effectiveness and that nonverbal approaches work more effectively. A meta-analysis of different treatment approaches found that massage and touch therapy were more effective than other approaches for reducing verbal aggression (Watt et al., 2019). This meta-analysis also found that these approaches, along with outdoor activities, were more effective than some medications for treating aggression. It is interesting to consider these findings along with the research findings showing that physical touch reduces the level of stress in dogs known to be associated with barking (Mariti et al., 2018; McGowan et al. 2018).

Research also supports that behavioral approaches emphasizing classical conditioning can be used to both address barking in dogs and agitated behaviors in humans. For example, research has supported that classical conditioning can reduce barking in animal shelters (Payne & Assemi, 2017). In addition, classical conditioning is severely impaired but is still possible even in more severe cases of Alzheimer's Disease (Woodruff-Pak et al., 1996). Based on this research, there is reason to expect that basic classical conditioning approaches can be used effectively for addressing agitated behaviors in dementia, much in the same way they can help control vocalizations in nonhuman animals. Research on specific behavioral approaches has been severely limited, but what is out there has shown some promising effects.

There are also other approaches shown to work on barking in dogs that may also have a helpful effect on reducing agitated behaviors in humans. Pheromones have been shown to help reduce barking and other evidence of increased stress among dogs in an animal shelter (Tod et al., 2005). This indicates the degree to which pheromones help reduce the types of stressors that lead to barking. What is particularly interesting here is that there have been suggestions among professionals. However, no formal research has shown that pheromones might also help decrease agitated behaviors associated with dementia in humans (Liu & Howard, 2015).

When considering the similarities between barking in dogs and agitated behaviors among dementia patients, it is interesting to consider research showing that dog visits have decreased agitated behaviors among dementia patients in nursing homes (Olsen et al., 2016). This research has shown the helpful impact of dogs on agitated patients, but the reason why has not been clear. It is interesting to consider that there may be a level of comfort between two individuals trying to maneuver through a world that has periods of intense emotional distress and for whom both need a sense of social support and connectedness without the specificity of verbal communication.

References

Darwin, C. (1872). *The Expression of Emotion in Man and Animals*. London: John Murray.

Feil, N. (2014). Validation therapy with late-onset dementia populations. *Caregiving in Dementia: Research and Applications*, *1*, 199–218.

Gouzoules, H., & Gouzoules, S. (1989). Design features and developmental modification of pigtail macaque, Macaca nemestrina, agonistic screams. *Animal Behaviour*, *37*, 383–401. https://doi.org/10.1016/0003-3472(89)90086-9

Jégh-Czinege, N., Faragó, T., & Pongrácz, P. (2020). A bark of its own kind–the acoustics of 'annoying'dog barks suggests a specific attention-evoking effect for humans. *Bioacoustics*, *29*(2), 210–225.68. https://doi.org/10.1080/09524622.2019.1576147

Kello, C. T., Bella, S. D., Médé, B., & Balasubramaniam, R. (2017). Hierarchical temporal structure in music, speech and animal vocalizations: Jazz is like a conversation, humpbacks sing like hermit thrushes. *Journal of The Royal Society Interface*, *14*(135), 20170231. https://doi.org/10.1098/rsif.2017.0231

Liu, K., & Howard, R. J. (2015). Could pheromones have a place in the management of agitation in dementia? *International Journal of Geriatric Psychiatry*, *2*(30), 219–220. http://dx.doi.org/10.1002%2Fgps.4210

Mariti, C., Carlone, B., Protti, M., Diverio, S., & Gazzano, A. (2018). Effects of petting before a brief separation from the owner on dog behavior and physiology: A pilot study. *Journal of Veterinary Behavior*, *27*, 41–46. https://doi.org/10.1016/j.jveb.2018.07.003

Maskeliunas, R., Raudonis, V., & Damasevicius, R. (2018). Recognition of emotional vocalizations of canine. *Acta Acustica United with Acustica*, *104*(2), 304–314. https://doi.org/10.3813/AAA.919173

McGowan, R. T., Bolte, C., Barnett, H. R., Perez-Camargo, G., & Martin, F. (2018). Can you spare 15 min? The measurable positive impact of a 15-min petting session on shelter dog well-being. *Applied Animal Behaviour Science*, *203*, 42–54.

McGreevy, P. (2004). Ethology of barking–why do dogs bark. In: *Proceedings of the National Urban Animal Management Conference, Adelaide* (pp. 9–10).

Minyo, M., & Judge, K. (2020). Unmet needs and behavioral expressions: The perspective of individuals with mild to moderate dementia. *Innovation in Aging, 4*(Suppl 1), 881. https://doi.org/10.1093%2Fgeroni%2Figaa057.3254

Olsen, C., Pedersen, I., Bergland, A., Enders-Slegers, M. J., Patil, G., & Ihlebæk, C. (2016). Effect of animal-assisted interventions on depression, agitation and quality of life in nursing home residents suffering from cognitive impairment or dementia: A cluster randomized controlled trial. *International Journal of Geriatric Psychiatry, 31*(12), 1312–1321. https://doi.org/10.1002/gps.4436

Payne, S. W., & Assemi, K. S. (2017). An evaluation of respondent conditioning procedures to decrease barking in an animal shelter. *Pet Behaviour Science*, (3), 19–24. https://doi.org/10.21071/pbs.v0i3.5858

Pérez-Espinosa, H., Reyes-Meza, V., Aguilar-Benitez, E., & Sanzón-Rosas, Y. M. (2018). Automatic individual dog recognition is based on the acoustic properties of its bark. *Journal of Intelligent & Fuzzy Systems, 34*(5), 3273–3280. https://doi.org/10.3233/JIFS-169509

Petrovsky, D. V., Sefcik, J. S., Hodgson, N. A., & Gitlin, L. N. (2020). Harsh communication: Characteristics of caregivers and persons with dementia. *Aging & Mental Health, 24*(10), 1709–1716. https://doi.org/10.1080/13607863.2019.1667296

Pongrácz, P., Molnár, C., & Miklósi, Á. (2010). Barking in family dogs: An ethological approach. *The Veterinary Journal, 183*(2), 141–147. https://doi.org/10.1016/j.tvjl.2008.12.010

Pongrácz, P., Lenkei, R., Marx, A., & Faragó, T. (2017). Should I whine, or should I bark? Qualitative and quantitative differences between the vocalizations of dogs with and without separation-related symptoms. *Applied Animal Behaviour Science, 196*, 61–68. https://doi.org/10.1016/j.applanim.2017.07.002

Ravignani, A., Dalla Bella, S., Falk, S., Kello, C. T., Noriega, F., & Kotz, S. A. (2019). Rhythm in speech and animal vocalizations: A cross-species perspective. *Annals of the New York Academy of Sciences, 1453*(1), 79. https://doi.org/10.1111%2Fnyas.14166

Ruusila, V., & Pesonen, M. (2004, January). Interspecific cooperation in human (Homo sapiens) hunting: The benefits of a barking dog (Canis familiaris). In: *Annales Zoologici Fennici* (pp. 545–549). Finnish Zoological and Botanical Publishing Board. https://www.jstor.org/stable/23735938

Scheumann, M., Hasting, A. S., Zimmermann, E., & Kotz, S. A. (2017). Human novelty response to emotional animal vocalizations: Effects of phylogeny and familiarity. *Frontiers in Behavioral Neuroscience, 11*, 204. https://doi.org/10.3389/fnbeh.2017.00204

Testad, I., Auer, S., Mittelman, M., Ballard, C., Fossey, J., Donabauer, Y., & Aarsland, D. (2010). Nursing home structure and association with agitation and use of psychotropic drugs in nursing home residents in three countries: Norway, Austria and England. *International Journal of Geriatric Psychiatry, 25*(7), 725–731. https://doi.org/10.1002/gps.2414

Tod, E., Brander, D., & Waran, N. (2005). Efficacy of dog appeasing pheromone in reducing stress and fear related behaviour in shelter dogs. *Applied Animal Behaviour Science, 93*(3–4), 295–308. https://doi.org/10.1016/j.applanim.2005.01.007

Watt, J. A., Goodarzi, Z., Veroniki, A. A., Nincic, V., Khan, P. A., Ghassemi, M., … & Straus, S. E. (2019). Comparative efficacy of interventions for aggressive and agitated behaviors in dementia: A systematic review and network meta-analysis. *Annals of Internal Medicine, 171*(9), 633–642. https://doi.org/10.7326/M19-0993

Woodruff-Pak, D. S., Papka, M., Romano, S., & Li, Y. T. (1996). Eyeblink classical conditioning in Alzheimer's disease and cerebrovascular dementia. *Neurobiology of Aging, 17*(4), 505–512. https://doi.org/10.1016/0197-4580(96)00070-X

Yin, S. (2002). A new perspective on barking in dogs (Canis familaris.). *Journal of Comparative Psychology, 116*(2), 189. https://doi.org/10.1037/0735-7036.116.2.189

Yin, S., & McCowan, B. (2004). Barking in domestic dogs: Context specificity and individual identification. *Animal Behaviour, 68*(2), 343–355. https://doi.org/10.1016/j.anbehav.2003.07.016

7 Ethological Research as an Alternative to Experimentation

Introduction

Comparative psychopathology presents a different way of defining and understanding psychological disorders. So far, this book has focused on differences in utilizing psychological research of all kinds to understand constructs and processes essential for a more comprehensive understanding of psychopathology. Throughout this book, we have described research other than clinical research as both experimental and observational. Experimental research is the research approach most often referenced when discussing psychological research. This chapter will address the observational approach to research, or ethological research, that makes up a significant portion of comparative psychology research. It is a research approach whose findings should make up a large portion of what is used in comparative psychopathology. It could offer an additional avenue to expand on what is used in comparative psychopathology.

This chapter will explore an alternative to experimentation as the primary research method in psychology. Experimentation is based on control of variables and group comparisons. It has been the predominant approach to psychology research since its beginning over 100 years ago. However, in the field of comparative psychology, ethology has been a method rivaling experimentation as the primary research method. In recent decades, ethology has been used even more and applied to studying human psychology. These are reasons why ethology is worth considering as a major component of research in the field of comparative psychopathology.

Ethology as an important addition to understanding psychological disorders has been proposed for some time. Over 40 years ago, Eibl-Eibesfeldt (1979) proposed that ethology has more of a place in human psychological research, not only for incorporating observation into understanding human psychology but also for more of a focus on behavioral aspects associated with survival. Fox and Fleising (1976) also addressed the benefit of ethological research for expanding on the evolutionary constructs used in

DOI: 10.4324/9781003408918-8

psychology. These authors presented the benefit of ethology for expanding psychology's knowledge base, including the knowledge base for understanding psychological disorders and advancing psychology with a more comprehensive incorporation of all evolutionary principles.

Taking a comprehensive view of incorporating all branches of evolution into a field of study means incorporating social evolution and other types of evolution. Since psychology is not a biological science, social evolution would have more relevance than biological or genetic evolution principles. This is the basis behind the field of "evolutionary psychology," which emphasizes the role that social behaviors have in helping individuals survive and adapt. Survival and social instincts are biological constructs that serve as the basis for why individuals adapt to environmental changes. However, how those adaptions function is primarily related to social and cultural means rather than genetic ones (Richerson et al., 2021). Ethological research is a significant contributor to understanding cultural and social evolution (Bender, 2021; Eibl-Eibesfeldt, 2014; Henrich & McElreath, 2003; Testard, Tremblay, & Platt, 2021), and its incorporation into a comprehensive study of psychopathology would be an important step at including these branches of evolutionary principles into this field.

History of Experimentation in Psychology Research

Experimentation has been the primary mode of psychology research since the late 19th century. During this period, psychology established itself as a scientific discipline, aiming to adopt the empirical methods and rigor of the natural sciences. Influenced by the advances in physiology and physics, psychologists sought to apply experimental methods to understand the human mind's and behavior's complexities. Academic material on using experimental methods to study concepts relevant to psychology dates back to 1853 and earlier (Wixted, 2020).

Wilhelm Wundt, often considered the founder of experimental psychology, established the first psychological laboratory in Leipzig, Germany, in 1879 (Diriwächter, 2021). Wundt and his students conducted controlled experiments, employing introspection and objective measurement to study various psychological processes. It is interesting to consider that Wundt's accomplishment was primarily in advancing the importance of experimental psychology rather than any particular experimental finding (Danziger, 2020). He is known more for establishing the scientific method as a major aspect of psychological research rather than for any particular psychology theory.

Behavioral psychology, advanced in the early 20th century, further solidified experimentation as the dominant approach in psychology. Behaviorists such as John B. Watson and B.F. Skinner emphasized the study of observable behaviors and advocated for rigorous experimental methods to understand the principles of learning and behavior. In the 1950s, a group of psychologists at Harvard, including B.F. Skinner considerably advanced the importance of experimental psychology, with particular importance placed on the operational definition of variables (Verhaegh, 2021). The use of experiments allowed for manipulating variables, establishing cause-and-effect relationships and developing theories grounded in empirical evidence. As psychology grew as a scientific discipline, experimentation became increasingly valued for its ability to provide systematic and replicable findings, leading to its widespread adoption as the primary approach in psychological research.

Experimentation and Its Role in Psychology

Experiments in human psychology research typically follow a systematic and controlled approach to investigate various aspects of human behavior and cognition. This system has been both a source of strength for research and a source of weakness. Its structure is presented as a reason why solid conclusions can be made based on results. This same structure is identified as a weakness as this often removes experiments from naturalistic environments.

Here is the approach typically taken in psychological experiments. Firstly, researchers begin by formulating a research question they want to address. Once they establish a research question, the next step is to develop an educated guess, otherwise known as a "hypothesis." Researchers then design an experiment to test this hypothesis and collect relevant data. Experimental studies often involve the manipulation of independent variables, which are factors that researchers can control or manipulate, to observe their effects on dependent variables, which are the variables being measured or observed. This manipulation is typically done by creating different experimental conditions or groups.

Once the experimental design is established, participants are recruited and assigned randomly to different groups or conditions. This random assignment helps ensure that any observed differences between groups are due to the manipulated independent variable rather than pre-existing differences between participants. Researchers then collect data through various methods such as observations, questionnaires, cognitive tasks, or physiological measurements. During the experiment, researchers carefully control extraneous variables, which are factors that could potentially influence the results but are not of interest in the study, to minimize their impact and enhance the internal validity of the study.

After data collection, researchers analyze the data using statistical techniques to determine if there are significant differences between groups or conditions. This analysis helps draw conclusions and evaluate the hypothesis. Additionally, ethical considerations play a crucial role in the experimental process, as researchers must ensure that participants' rights, privacy, and well-being are protected throughout the study. Overall, experimental studies in human psychology provide a rigorous and systematic approach to understanding human behavior and cognition, allowing researchers to draw reliable conclusions about cause-and-effect relationships between variables.

Limitations of Experimental Approach Used in Psychology

Over the past century, experimentation has been the primary model researchers have used to learn about psychological processes. Psychological research relies heavily on experimentation to investigate various aspects of human behavior and cognition. It has obtained a privileged status within psychology (Diener et al., 2022). While experiments are an invaluable tool in this field, researchers must consider several inherent limitations.

Many psychological experiments take place in controlled laboratory settings. While these environments allow researchers to manipulate variables and maintain consistency, they may not accurately reflect real-world situations (Nastase et al., 2020). Participants' behavior in a controlled setting might differ from their behavior in natural settings, leading to a lack of ecological validity. Psychology experiments provide very important information, but there is a high degree to which those results seem artificial and manufactured. Without a reliance on the natural environment, there is a sense that the results do not always relate to the real world. This often limits how much researchers can comfortably determine what results say about how psychological variables are interconnected (Gile, 1998).

Psychological experiments often rely on small and selective samples of participants, which may not represent the diversity of the larger population. Consequently, the generalizability of findings to the broader population can be limited (Maxwell, 2021). Furthermore, certain participant characteristics, such as age, gender, and cultural background, can influence responses and introduce confounding variables.

Conducting experiments can be time-consuming, and researchers often have limited resources and deadlines to meet. As a result, experiments may have to be conducted within relatively short timeframes, which might not capture certain psychological processes' full complexity and dynamics. This has also limited the types of settings where research can be conducted and has caused difficulties with researchers with less access to resources, often leaving them out of the process (Marston & GoPaul, 2019; Marston & GoPaul, 2020).

In experiments, participants are often asked to perform specific tasks that may not fully represent the complexity and variability of real-world cognitive processes. Simplified tasks can overlook crucial factors and fail to capture human behavior and decision-making nuances in complex, everyday situations. Psychological research through experimentation often does not capture the reality of how people live their daily lives (Holleman et al., 2020)

Experimenters' biases and expectations can inadvertently influence the outcomes of studies (Morawski, 2019). Unintentional cues, subtle nonverbal behavior, or unintentional reinforcement can all introduce bias into the experimental process, affecting participants' responses and distorting the results. This, again, is a characteristic of the more manufactured setting involved with experiments. Although researchers have to be careful not to allow their observational techniques to impact results, there is much less impact of researchers' bias associated with ethology than experimentation (Tuyttens et al., 2016).

Replicating experiments is essential for establishing the reliability and validity of experimental findings (Fabrigar et al., 2020). However, replication studies are not always conducted due to time, resources, and publication bias. Without replication, it becomes difficult to determine the generalizability and robustness of experimental findings. Replicability is not stronger or better with ethology, but it is an approach that considers alternatives to replication for generalizability (Nawroth & Gygax, 2023).

Some psychological phenomena cannot be directly manipulated due to ethical or practical constraints. For example, researchers cannot ethically manipulate variables such as trauma, early life experiences, or certain neurological conditions. These limitations restrict the ability to investigate certain aspects of human behavior through experimental means. Ethology research allows for observation of the phenomena and provides a structured and objective alternative to concerns about manipulating variables.

Human behavior is influenced by a wide range of individual differences, including personality traits, cognitive abilities, and past experiences. Experiments often aim to identify general patterns and average effects, which may overlook the significant variability and unique characteristics of individuals. In ethology research, the focus is more general, and there is not necessarily the case that targeting variables and their effect is the goal. This can make explaining how variables are related difficult. Still, the complexities of human life make it likely that explaining how variables are related and what variables have what impact should be challenging. Ethology research, in this way, provides a means of investigating phenomena in ways more consistent with the complex ways the human and animal worlds likely work.

While experiments are a valuable tool in psychological research, they have limitations. Researchers must be mindful of these limitations and consider alternative methods, such as naturalistic observations, field studies, and qualitative research, to complement and enhance their understanding of human behavior. By employing a diverse range of research methods, psychologists can gain a more comprehensive and nuanced understanding of the complexities of the human mind and behavior. Since earning a more comprehensive and nuanced understanding of psychological disorders has been the goal of comparative psychopathology expressed throughout this book, it is valuable and important to consider other research approaches to emphasize.

Ethological Research as an Alternative to Experimentation

Given the limitations of the experimental approach used in psychology it is worthwhile to consider other alternatives to studying behaviors. One alternative approach used in human and nonhuman animal studies is the ethological approach. It is an approach that has been used for studying nonhuman animals for many decades and has, in more recent decades, been applied to human psychology research. Ethological research offers an alternative approach to studying behavior in psychology, particularly when focusing on nonhuman animals (e.g. Pearce & Wang, 2019). This approach emphasizes naturalistic observations (Mobbs et al., 2021). It puts it more in conjunction with what should be expected from a comparative psychology perspective for understanding psychopathology.

Ethological research focuses on observation rather than experimentation. Researchers using this approach do not manipulate variables but observe the impact of different variables as they occur in natural settings. There is a real need for this type of research emphasized more in psychology, as research focusing on observations rather than manipulations seems to have been lost (Bonetto et al., 2023). Focusing on psychological processes as they occur in the natural environments gives researchers the opportunity to witness how variables truly impact other variables rather than how they impact variables when certain conditions are manufactured. This would go a long way to really understanding what is happening when it comes to investigating the causes and maintenance of psychological disorders.

Rather than relying solely on experiments, ethological research delves into the natural habitats and social contexts of animals to gain a deeper understanding of their behavior. This approach emphasizes observation, documentation, and analysis of animals in their natural environments, allowing for a more ecologically valid and comprehensive understanding of their behavior (Peters et al., 2015). Ethological research embraces the complexity and individuality of animal behavior, recognizing that it is shaped by various factors such as social dynamics, ecological constraints, and evolutionary adaptations. By studying animals in their natural contexts, ethological research can provide insights into the natural behaviors and interactions that may be difficult or unethical to replicate in a controlled laboratory setting. It allows for exploring behavioral patterns, social structures, and environmental influences, contributing to a more nuanced understanding of animal behavior and its ecological significance.

Comparing the merits of ethological research and experimentation in the field of animal behavior is not a matter of one being inherently better than the other but rather a recognition of their distinct advantages and limitations. Ethological research offers a unique perspective by studying animals in their natural environments, allowing for a deeper understanding of their behavior within the context of their ecological and evolutionary adaptations. It provides valuable insights into social dynamics, natural selection pressures, and the intricate relationships between animals and their habitats (De Paepe et al., 2019).

Rather than focus on experiments in very controlled environments, ethological research captures the richness and complexity of real-world behaviors. It offers a holistic approach that acknowledges the diversity and variability within species. Experimentation, with its controlled settings and manipulations, allows for more identification of cause-and-effect relationships. As such, experiments provide valuable insights into underlying mechanisms and offer a level of control often not feasible in the wild (Modliński & Gladden, 2021). What is not knowable in experiments is the degree to which removing the naturalistic setting removes actual variables that also impact behaviors.

Ethological research has traditionally been considered a branch of biology that focuses on studying animal behavior in their natural environments. In recent decades, it has also been seen as a branch of other areas, including psychology, leadership studies (Cook et al., 2020), and economics (Shcherbakova, 2019). Ethologists spend significant time observing animals in their natural habitats. They carefully document behaviors such as feeding, mating, communication, and territoriality. Observational studies provide insights into the daily routines, social structures, and individual variations within a species. It is considered the observational path of research, in contrast to the experimental path emphasized throughout much of psychology's history.

Ethologists primarily use field studies to observe animal behavior. Field research involves conducting observations and experiments in the animals' natural environments. Researchers may track individuals or study entire populations. By gathering data directly from the field, ethologists can understand how animals adapt to their specific habitats and respond to environmental changes. They frequently compare the behavior of different species to identify common patterns or evolutionary trends. By studying a range of species, researchers can gain insights into the origins and functions of behaviors across the animal kingdom.

When analyzing data collected during field studies, ethologists primarily employ statistical tools and data analysis techniques to make sense of the vast amount of behavioral data they collect. They use descriptive statistics, correlations, regression analysis, and other quantitative methods to identify significant relationships and patterns in the data. Statistics are the common denominator between experimental and ethology research. There is still an emphasis on using statistics as the objective means of making conclusions in ethology research.

Ethology provides an objective means of understanding how variables in the natural environment impact behaviors and functioning. Although the focus is not on controlling variables that are not being studied, as is the case with extraneous variables in experimentation, there is still a focus on structured means of collecting observational data. Statistical analysis provides the objective means by which the data is analyzed and interpreted. In these ways, ethology as an alternative to experimentation still keeps comparative psychopathology as an objective and structured approach to better understanding psychological disorders.

Human Ethology Research

When considering approaches for researching the causes of human psychopathology, it is helpful to consider the benefits of ethology over the prominent experimental approach. Ethology focuses on observing animals in their natural habitats, allowing researchers to study behavior in a context that closely resembles the animals' everyday lives. This approach provides valuable insights into the complex interactions between animals and their environment, including social dynamics, territorial behavior, mating rituals, and foraging strategies. Psychopathology as a field would likely benefit from more naturalistic studies on how variables like this impact the development and maintenance of psychological disorders.

By studying animals in their natural settings, ethologists observe behaviors that may be difficult to replicate in a laboratory setting. Ethology also considers the ecological and evolutionary factors that shape behavior providing a comprehensive understanding of how animals adapt and survive in their specific environments. This approach emphasizes a holistic view of animal behavior, acknowledging the intricate interplay between genetics, physiology, and environmental influences. In contrast, the experimental approach often isolates animals from their natural contexts, potentially leading to artificial behaviors and limited generalizability. While both approaches have their merits, the ethology approach offers a rich and ecologically valid framework for studying animal behavior.

Human ethology relies upon principles and methods from ethology to investigate human behavior. It seeks to understand human behavior in the context of our evolutionary heritage, considering the adaptive functions, social dynamics, and ecological influences that shape our actions. Human ethologists rely on observational methods to study behavior in naturalistic settings. They carefully observe and document human interactions and behaviors in real-world contexts, aiming to capture the richness and complexity of human behavior as it naturally unfolds.

Human ethologists often employ ethnographic methods, such as participant observation and in-depth interviews, to gain a deep understanding of cultural practices, beliefs, and social norms. These qualitative methods allow researchers to uncover the underlying meanings and motivations of human behavior. Field studies provide valuable insights into the cultural, social, and environmental factors influencing human behavior.

Human ethologists compare human behavior with other species to identify similarities, differences, and shared evolutionary roots. By studying nonhuman animals, researchers can gain insights into specific behaviors' evolutionary origins and functions, shedding light on our behavior as a species. It also places a strong emphasis on studying social interactions and relationships. Researchers investigate various aspects of social behavior, including cooperation, competition, dominance, altruism, and mate choice. They explore how social factors influence our behavior and shape our social structures.

History of Ethology and the Study of Psychopathology

What all the material covered in this chapter supports is that ethology offers some benefits compared to experimental methods. It is best to consider ethology as an alternative approach to psychological research rather than a superior method. Its emphasis on naturalistic observation is one strength, while its limited ability to control variables is one weakness compared to experimentation.

There is a solid argument to be made that ethology represents a strong alternative to consider for studying psychopathology. Its strengths fit quite well with what experimentation does not offer when studying psychological disorders. This includes emphasizing disorders as they occur in the natural environment instead of controlled laboratory settings.

Ethological research used for studying psychopathology has been implemented since the beginning of psychology as a distinct science. Ivan Pavlov, the founder of classical conditioning as a psychological concept, discussed experimental neurosis and used animal observations to show the process by which psychological disorders develop and progress (Windholz, 1991). Pavlov's concept of experimental neurosis involved inducing a state of confusion or conflict in an animal subject by presenting it with contradictory or ambiguous signals. The animal could no longer predict the outcome of a situation based on the stimuli it received. For instance, the dog might hear a bell (a conditioned stimulus) and sometimes receive food (an unconditioned stimulus), but other times it would not. This inconsistency can lead to a condition similar to neurosis in humans, characterized by abnormal behavior, anxiety, and confusion. This concept provided significant insights into understanding human neuroses. It suggested that mental disorders in humans might also be the result of situations or environments that are inconsistent, unpredictable, or contradictory.

Pavlov's work was followed by Joseph Wolpe, who expanded on the concept of experimental neurosis (Wolpe, 1952). Wolpe built upon Pavlov's original concept. While Pavlov induced experimental neurosis in dogs using contradictory signals, Wolpe introduced a more ethical and practical method that involved cats. His work involved conditioning cats to associate a harmless stimulus with an unpleasant situation. For example, he would present a sound to the cats while simultaneously giving them mild electric shocks. Over time, the cats became so conditioned to this pattern that they would show signs of anxiety and fear at the sound, even in the absence of the shocks. These symptoms mirrored those of neurosis in humans.

Wolpe's work on experimental neurosis is an excellent example of how behavioral observations of nonhuman animals led directly to a treatment model for humans. Wolpe's most significant contribution to clinical psychology is the development of systematic desensitization, developed as a response to this induced fear. Systematic desensitization involves gradually exposing a subject to the fear-inducing stimulus in a controlled and safe environment while teaching them to use relaxation techniques to counteract the anxiety. This process aims to break the association between the stimulus and the fear response. His work is an excellent example of ethological psychology research directly impacting clinical psychology.

The most famous example of ethological research used to understand psychopathology is Howard Lindell and the "Behavior Farm" at Cornell University (Kirk & Ramsden, 2018). Interestingly, in the Kirk and Ramsden article, they even reference Lidell and colleagues using the term "comparative psychopathology" to describe their work. Whereas Pavlov and Wolpe conducted their work based primarily on behavioral observations associated with ethology, they still conducted those observations in structured laboratories under some controlled conditions. On the other hand, Liddell created an actual farm where psychopathology and its development could be observed as nonhuman animals lived their lives. Liddell developed a laboratory where the study of nonhuman animals, including pigs and sheep, was used to understand the development of psychological disorders. Liddell did this to bring psychology more in line with biology and medicine, which is why comparative psychopathology has been proposed as an important field throughout this book.

Reviewing the history of ethology applied to the study of psychological disorders reveals the benefits of this approach. Studying behaviors in a naturalistic environment allows for opportunities to study more factors impacting disorders. Pavlov supported this by identifying factors associated with classical conditioning impacting neuroses. Behavioral observations allow for observations of psychopathological development separate from whether the individuals meet formalized diagnostic criteria. Pavlov's and Wolpe's work had more of an influence on the development of the diagnostic criteria for conditions like depression and anxiety rather than those criteria directly in their research. Ethological research also allowed for studying psychopathology and the factors impacting its development and maintenance as part of the daily lives experienced by animals. Psychopathology, in the case of Liddell's farm, was only part of what was happening in these individual's lives rather than the sole focus of what was happening in their lives. This represents potential strengths for using ethological research as an alternative to or companion to psychological experimentation.

Human Ethology and Comparative Psychopathology

In the 2006 article on the need to expand psychological research, Paul Rozin summarized well the potential benefit of giving more attention to observational research like human ethology:

> "Psychology would profit from paying greater attention to describing and explaining what people do, an endeavor that would perhaps be facilitated by a focus on the domains of daily life."
>
> (Rozin, 2006)

Ethological approaches have been proposed as an important addition to understanding psychopathology. This comes from its importance in studying psychological constructs across species and in understanding psychological constructs specifically for humans. This approach is called "human ethology," and there is at least one academic journal ("Human Ethology Bulletin") specifically focused on this topic and one professional organization specifically dedicated to this field ("International Society of Human Ethology").

Human ethology research shows a great deal that helps expand our understanding of psychological disorders. Here are some examples of human ethology research on psychological disorders:

- During clinical interviews, depressed patients show signs of "arrested flight." This reflects the triggering of the "fight-or-flight" response when escape ("flight") is hampered (Dixon, 1998).

- Observations of individuals with anxiety disorders show that anxiety often relates to the individual trying actively, either consciously or subconsciously, to escape an immediate threat (Coelho et al., 2023). This indicates that the difference between anxiety and depression could be that anxiety relates to an active attempt to escape a perceived threat, and depression relates to the individual recognizing, again, consciously or unconsciously, that escape is hampered.
- Individuals with schizophrenia do not suffer from an impoverishment of nonverbal behaviors but, rather, from an excess of nonverbal behaviors that are not consistent with what is happening in the person's environment. These behaviors are often consistent with what seems to be a misinterpretation of sensory input, especially olfactory input, and ritualized behaviors with no clear purpose (Manoel et al., 2021; Samokhvalov & Samokhvalova, 2011).
- Individuals with drug addiction disorders show a greater number of behaviors consistent with communicating a preference for keeping distance and a lower number of behaviors associated with maintaining group affiliation. This suggests that substance abuse problems may be correlated with individuals having a preference for being outside of any type of recognized social group (Verbitskaya et al., 2007).
- Lack of gaze, physical aversion, looking at one's own body rather than at others, taking things without asking, lack of sharing behaviors, and climbing were all behaviors distinguishing individuals with autism from individuals without autism. This included differentiating between individuals with autism from individuals with no diagnosed conditions and differentiating individuals with autism from individuals with intellectual disabilities (Pegoraro et al., 2014).

These examples show the benefits that ethology has for studying psychopathology. Not only do these research studies allow for observation to reveal behaviors and psychological constructs in their natural states, but they also show the benefit that observations can have for advancing diagnostics. Notice how the Pegoraro study relates to what psychologists can look for when observing behaviors to help with the differential autism diagnosis. Behavioral observations are often overlooked parts of psychological assessments and need to be more standardized for increased effectiveness (Newson et al., 2020). Ethological research provides a means for standardization and a means of more fully understanding the psychological disorders being diagnosed.

Summary

To be a comprehensive way of understanding psychological disorders, comparative psychopathology needs to have a relevant research approach. Incorporating research from all different areas means incorporating both experimental and observational research. There are solid reasons for concluding that psychology has tended to emphasize experimental research and comparative psychopathology as a new way of understanding and studying psychological disorders and can take the lead in incorporating observational research as well.

Ethology research emphasizes behavioral observations and is prominent throughout comparative psychology studies. Incorporating it more into the study of psychopathology than has been the case recently would help to give a more comprehensive view of this area. Ethology studies provide useful information for understanding more about the psychological constructs contributing to psychological disorders. It allows for more understanding of the natural environment in which these constructs exist and in which psychological disorders develop. Ethology research takes away the manufactured environments in which most experiments occur in exchange for the natural environment in which phenomena occur. In this way, ethology research is an addition to, and not a replacement for, what information experimental research offers.

References

Bender, N. (2021). Contribution of ethology to evolutionary medicine. *Ethology*, *127*(10), 821–826.

Bonetto, E., Guiller, T., & Adam-Troian, J. (2023). A lost idea in psychology: Observation as starting point for the scientific investigation of human behavior. *Human Ethology*, *38*(1), 8–16. https://doi.org/10.22330/he/38/008-016

Coelho, C. M., Araujo, A. S., Suttiwan, P., & Zsido, A. N. (2023). An ethologically based view into human fear. *Neuroscience & Biobehavioral Reviews*, *145*, 105017.

Cook, A. S., Zill, A., & Meyer, B. (2020). Observing leadership as behavior in teams and herds–An ethological approach to shared leadership research. *The Leadership Quarterly*, *31*(2), 101296.

Danziger, K. (2020). Wilhelm Wundt and the emergence of experimental psychology. In: *Companion to the History of Modern Science* (pp. 396–409). Routledge.

De Paepe, A. L., Williams, A. C. D. C., & Crombez, G. (2019). Habituation to pain: a motivational-ethological perspective. *Pain*, *160*(8), 1693–1697.

Diener, E., Northcott, R., Zyphur, M. J., & West, S. G. (2022). Beyond experiments. *Perspectives on Psychological Science*, *17*(4), 1101–1119.

Diriwächter, R. (2021). Remembering wilhelm wundt and the second leipzig school of psychology. *Human Arenas*, *4*, 5–19.

Dixon, A. K. (1998). Ethological strategies for defense in animals and humans: Their role in some psychiatric disorders. *British Journal of Medical Psychology*, *71*(4), 417–445.

Eibl-Eibesfeldt, I. (1979). Human ethology: Concepts and implications for the sciences of man. *Behavioral and Brain Sciences*, *2*(1), 1–26.

Eibl-Eibesfeldt, I. (2014). The comparative approach in human ethology. In: *Comparing Behavior* (pp. 43–65). Psychology Press.

Fabrigar, L. R., Wegener, D. T., & Petty, R. E. (2020). A validity-based framework for understanding replication in psychology. *Personality and Social Psychology Review*, *24*(4), 316–344.

Fox, R., & Fleising, U. (1976). Human ethology. *Annual Review of Anthropology, 5*(1), 265–288.

Holleman, G. A., Hooge, I. T., Kemner, C., & Hessels, R. S. (2020). The 'real-world approach' and its problems: A critique of ecological validity. *Frontiers in Psychology, 11*, 721.

Gile, D. (1998). Observational studies and experimental studies in the investigation of conference interpreting. *Target. International Journal of Translation Studies, 10*(1), 69–93.

Henrich, J., & McElreath, R. (2003). The evolution of cultural evolution. *Evolutionary Anthropology: Issues, News, and Reviews: Issues, News, and Reviews, 12*(3), 123–135.

Kirk, R. G., & Ramsden, E. (2018). Working across species down on the farm: Howard S. Liddell and the development of comparative psychopathology, c. 1923–1962. *History and Philosophy of the Life Sciences, 40*, 1–29.

Manoel, D., Makhlouf, M., Arayata, C. J., Sathappan, A., Da'as, S., Abdelrahman, D., & Saraiva, L. R. (2021). Deconstructing the mouse olfactory percept through an ethological atlas. *Current Biology, 31*(13), 2809–2818.

Marston, D., & Gopaul, M. (2019). Issues to consider for online doctoral candidates utilizing meta-analysis for dissertations. *International Journal of Online Graduate Education, 2*(1).

Marston, D., & Gopaul, M. (2020). Meta-synthesis: Issues to consider for online doctoral dissertations. *International Journal of Online Graduate Education, 3*(1).

Maxwell, J. A. (2021). Why qualitative methods are necessary for generalization. *Qualitative Psychology, 8*(1), 111.

Mobbs, D., Wise, T., Suthana, N., Guzmán, N., Kriegeskorte, N., & Leibo, J. Z. (2021). Promises and challenges of human computational ethology. *Neuron, 109*(14), 2224–2238.

Modliński, A., & Gladden, M. (2021). Applying ethology to design human-oriented technology. Experimental study on the signalling role of the labelling effect in technology's empowerment. *Human Technology, 17*(2), 164–189.

Morawski, J. (2019). The replication crisis: How might philosophy and theory of psychology be of use?. *Journal of Theoretical and Philosophical Psychology, 39*(4), 218.

Nastase, S. A., Goldstein, A., & Hasson, U. (2020). Keep it real: rethinking the primacy of experimental control in cognitive neuroscience. *NeuroImage, 222*, 117254.

Nawroth, C., & Gygax, L. (2023). The legislative, ethical, and conceptual importance of replicability in farm animal welfare science. *CABI Digital Library*. March 18, 2020. https://doi.org/10.31220/osf.io/ahspd

Newson, J. J., Hunter, D., & Thiagarajan, T. C. (2020). The heterogeneity of mental health assessment. *Frontiers in Psychiatry, 11*, 76.

Pearce, P. L., & Wang, Z. (2019). Human ethology and tourists' photographic poses. *Annals of Tourism Research, 74*, 108–120.

Pegoraro, L. F., Setz, E. Z., & Dalgalarrondo, P. (2014). Ethological approach to autism spectrum disorders. *Evolutionary Psychology, 12*(1), 147470491401200116.

Peters, S. M., Pothuizen, H. H., & Spruijt, B. M. (2015). Ethological concepts enhance the translational value of animal models. *European Journal of Pharmacology, 759*, 42–50.

Richerson, P. J., Gavrilets, S., & de Waal, F. B. (2021). Modern theories of human evolution foreshadowed by Darwin's Descent of Man. *Science, 372*(6544), eaba3776.

Rozin, P. (2006). Domain denigration and process preference in academic psychology. *Perspectives on Psychological Science, 1*(4), 365–376. https://doi.org/10.1111/j.1745-6916.2006.00021.x

Samokhvalov, V. P., & Samokhvalova, O. E. (2011). Toward a Neuroethology of Schizophrenia: Findings from the Crimean Project. *Handbook of Schizophrenia Spectrum Disorders, Volume II: Phenotypic and Endophenotypic Presentations*, (pp. 121–164).

Shcherbakova, N. V. (2019). The role of biological and economic factors in urban population growth. *R-Economy, 5*(3), 103–114.

Testard, C., Tremblay, S., & Platt, M. (2021). From the field to the lab and back: Neuroethology of primate social behavior. *Current Opinion in Neurobiology, 68*, 76–83. https://doi.org/10.1016/j.conb.2021.01.005

Tuyttens, F. A., Stadig, L., Heerkens, J. L., Buijs, S., & Ampe, B. (2016). Opinion of applied ethologists on expectation bias, blinding observers and other debiasing techniques. *Applied Animal Behaviour Science, 181*, 27–33.

Verbitskaya, E. V., Krupitsky, E. M., Burakov, A., Tsoy-Podosenina, M. V., Egorova, V. Y., Bushara, N., & Vekovischeva, O. Y. (2007). Nonverbal behavior of human addicts: Multimetric analysis. *Addictive Behaviors, 32*(10), 2260–2267.

Verhaegh, S. (2021). Psychological operationisms at Harvard: Skinner, Boring, and Stevens. *Journal of the History of the Behavioral Sciences, 57*(2), 194–212.

Windholz, G. (1991). Schilder and Pavlov's theory of higher nervous activity: A critique and apologia. *Integrative Physiological and Behavioral Science, 26*, 248–258.

Wixted, J. T. (2020). The forgotten history of signal detection theory. *Journal of Experimental Psychology: Learning, Memory, and Cognition, 46*(2), 201–233.

Wolpe, J. (1952). Experimental neuroses as learned behaviour. *British Journal of Psychology, 43*(4), 243.

8   Zoos as Comparative Psychopathology Laboratories

Introduction

Comparative psychopathology presents a fuller understanding of psychological disorders and psychological change than is the case with other approaches to understanding psychopathology. Experimental and observational research serve alongside clinical research, along with archival and meta-analysis research methods, to show all the factors involved in the creation and continuation of psychological disorders. Our proposal is that comprehensive psychopathology is a stronger approach than others because it is more complete and covers all angles of understanding psychopathological processes.

Different schools of psychological thought have settings particularly associated with those schools. This is true of the schools associated with understanding psychopathology. Freud used the consulting room at a time when most information about psychopathology came from the medical hospitals (Schubart, 1989). Jung used psychiatric hospitals to delve into the depths of psychological disorders at a time when those settings were primarily used for "warehousing" patients (Clark, 1955). Pavlov and Skinner used their scientific laboratories. Aaron Beck and Albert Ellis, both major names in cognitive-behavior psychotherapy, developed their own institutes where they collected relevant data.

Comparative psychopathology, as we propose its approach throughout this book, uses data and theories from all those settings. It is comprehensive in that it uses research from all different types of settings. There are, however, certain research settings and approaches more aligned with comparative psychopathology than with other schools of psychopathology theories. In Chapter 7 we discussed ethological research. Environments allowing for this type of observational research, naturalistic settings in particular, are environments that most set comparative psychopathology apart from other schools of understanding psychopathology. These include natural environments, observing animal behaviors out in the wild, or settings designed to

DOI: 10.4324/9781003408918-9

recreate natural environments. In comparative psychopathology, observational studies make up a large part of the knowledge base and serve a larger role than is the case in other approaches to understanding psychological disorders.

Ethology research and other types of observational research serve a large role in comparative psychopathology. Comparative psychology research in natural environments includes jungles, forests, and even backyards (e.g., Ayala et al., 2022; Gamble et al., 2023). These types of natural studies serve an important role but have limitations (Kummrow & Brüne, 2018). Observing animals out in the wild is unpredictable and requires keeping track of animals whereabouts over large areas. It is also very difficult to control any aspect of the environment when observing animals in the wild (Janmaat, 2019). All these factors make relying on observational studies out in the wild difficult.

Zoos present a solid means of studying animal psychology (Fernandez & Martin, 2021; Hopper, 2017) and an alternative to ethology studies in the wild. They provide restricted environments where the location of animals is always known. Longitudinal studies fit particularly well in zoos as the animals are in one limited area over time and do not move about large areas like in the wild. They offer the opportunity for a true study of comparative psychology. There is a great deal of biodiversity in zoos and zoological parks (including aquatic parks) that allows for comparative studies of many different animal species (Spooner et al., 2023; Miranda et al., 2023). It not only allows for the study of differences in psychological functioning among members of the same species but also a study of the psychological functioning of members across different species.

Zoos offer a strong resource for obtaining information important for advancing the knowledge base needed for comparative psychopathology. They have contributed a great deal to peer-reviewed research in recent decades (Kögler et al., 2020). Evaluating the quantitative and qualitative contribution of zoos and aquaria to peer-reviewed science [*Journal of Zoo and Aquarium Research*, *8*(2), 124-132], in this chapter, we will look at what zoos have contributed to understanding psychopathology and what they offer for advancing the understanding of psychopathology. We present in this chapter the real benefits zoos offer for psychological research and, in particular, psychopathology research. They offer the opportunity to understand behaviors across species and study longitudinally how different psychological factors impact functioning. They present opportunities to understand human psychological constructs better by providing the opportunity to observe how those constructs exist and function in nonhuman animals and also understand the psychological needs of nonhuman animals better. Zoos present a real means of using observations to more fully understand what happens when individuals, human and nonhuman, go about their daily lives.

What we are not doing in this chapter is making the case for or against zoos. Our position is that since zoos exist, the field of psychology should make use of what they offer. We realize that there are strong cases to be made for and against their existence. There are many positives about zoos and what they offer for both human and nonhuman animals (Greenwell et al., 2023; Learmonth, 2020). Zoos offer an opportunity for people to see how animals live and to understand them better. They offer humans the opportunity to understand the importance of conservation and taking care of the land better. When you have the chance to see up close who is depending on the land, we sometimes trample on, it is clearer why we have to protect it.

Although zoos offer a great deal of positives, there are negatives associated with zoos. They keep animals in captivity and limited spaces (Clay & Visseren-Hamakers, 2022). Very few zoos use cages, which was the case decades ago, and most provide animals with wide spaces to roam. They also provide settings that are very similar to animals' natural environments and that are much safer. Even so, animals in zoos are still confined and are not living truly free lives. Many argue that there is no way to compensate with safety and security for the loss of a truly free life. There is certainly value in this argument, and it is our position that the very least researchers and professionals need to do is make sure that there is sufficient value in what zoos offer, including what they offer to understand psychological functioning in human and nonhuman animals, to make the weaknesses worthwhile.

Howard Liddell's Behavior Farm

Although not technically a zoo, Liddell's "Behavior Farm" is possibly the best early example of how a restricted environment could be used to understand human and nonhuman psychopathology. He was the first to use the term "comparative psychopathology," and his use of this "farm" earned him the title of the "Father of Experimental Psychopathology in America" (Block, 1963). His work in 1936 was considered to be the leading research setting studying mental illness from a comparative psychology perspective and would remain that way for several decades (Broadhurst, 1960). Riddell was building on the concept of "experimental neurosis" presented by Pavlov (discussed in earlier chapters of the book).

What Lidell did nearly 100 years ago was show the way that facilities like zoos could be used for observing the development and maintenance of psychological disorders. Lidell used Pavlovian techniques to create pathology in different animal species and also studied the role of different interventions used for improving those pathological states. Lydell was open about his goal of creating the closest version of psychological disorders that could be created in nonhuman animal species. Although his purposeful creation of psychological disorders in animals may not be acceptable today, his work showed the benefits of a residential setting, where animals lived and where they could be observed frequently and even constantly throughout every day, in understanding psychological disorders.

Kirk and Ramsden (2018) provided a very good summary of Liddell's work. He started his behavior farm in 1923 and continued there until 1962. It was also known as the Cornell University Behavior Farm. There were 110 acres, and its purpose was to allow deviations from normal behaviors in animals to be studied. It was described as a place where the natural world was contained to allow behavioral study under controlled conditions. Its aim was to establish stable experiments and observational studies of neuroses for each animal species. This would serve as a tool for developing new psychological theories for human psychopathology. Animals living on the farm included dogs, rats, pigs, sheep, and goats. There was an experimental laboratory on the premises, but mainly, the animals roamed freely in controlled pastures and woodlands. Sheep were soon chosen as the main species because they frequently give birth to twins of the same sex. This allows for a clear pairing of experimental and control groups. In addition, wool and mutton from the sheep helped raise money for the farm's work.

Liddell began his research by examining how physiological differences affect animal learning and intelligence. He studied a large number of animals to address the impact of physical and environmental factors on behaviors. He did a large amount of work on studying the impact of thyroid deficiencies by studying groups of sheep who had thyroids and those that had their thyroids removed. He studied the physiological impact of thyroid absence on physical factors (Liddell, 1923b, 1925a) and on maze learning (Liddell, 1925b, 1926).

When Liddell started his work, he built on Pavlov's work by studying classical conditioning and saw psychopathology as primarily a physiological process. As his work with animals progressed, he soon saw that the scientific approach emphasizing conditional responses as purely physical phenomena was no longer adequate. He concluded that physiology alone could not explain the differences in learning and intelligence among the groups of animals he studied (Liddell, 1927).

As Liddell worked to study the impact of thyroid insufficiency in animals, he developed elaborate mazes to investigate animal intelligence and learning. He set out to study differences in how well and how quickly the sheep navigated through the mazes. What Liddell found, however, was that the physiological hypotheses he put forth to explain the differences between how the sheep ran these mazes could not explain adequately the differences between the groups. His conclusions (Liddell, 1954) over the decades that the behavior farm operated was that individual differences were what determined how, why, and how well the sheep ran through the mazes and changed the goals between individuals for why they were running through the mazes. He spent much of the decades working to define what factors accounted for these individual differences.

Lidell also concluded that the relationships between the researchers and the sheep were a prominent factor in the differences between the sheep. These researchers had not been just passive observers watching how and why the sheep ran the mazes but had become a major factor impacting the sheep's behaviors. He concluded that when the researchers implemented steps to create conditioned responses they in turn created traumatic environments for the animals. These was real changed measured in the context of the types of relationships these researchers had with the animals. He went on to focus much of his studies not only on individual differences but also relationships and their impact on conditional responses. He provides a large amount of research over the decades showing the often-complex interactions between individuals and their social and physical environment in the development of pathological behaviors.

From his work on animals and the mazes, along with other work on the farm, Liddell concluded that the conditioned reflex described by Pavlov is not exclusively related to learning and intelligence but is, rather, the "emotional context of behavior" (Liddell, 1954). He saw in the process of individuals developing responses to their environments complexity that showed the many different ways and intense ways individuals respond to what happens to them. This went a long way past the primarily physiological and straightforward these reflexes, often seen as the very bases of behaviors, had been viewed until then. His work on the farm led Liddell to write at one point. "The primitive forces of man's emotions are more dangerous and more devastating the nuclear fission" (Liddell, 1954). He wrote this in a landmark Science article, summarizing his work on neuroses induced in sheep, describing how irrational emotional behavior originates and how it could be prevented.

As Liddell witnessed the impact of emotions, relationships, and environmental factors on pathology he turned from a primary focus on experimentation to ethology. For him, ethology was a better method than others for understanding the complexities of how anxiety and neurosis relate to an animal's physical surroundings and social environment. He relied on ethology as a way of using observations to see what sort of patterns pathological behaviors followed in the animals on his farm. By doing this he moved away from experimentation where environments were manipulated and looked more at what happened in the environment, and how it impacted the animals. This included observations of how the animals interacted with the researchers and how the animals responded to what the researchers did. Taking this approach allowed him to present a large number of works over the years that showed the historical continuity of nervous behaviors where those behaviors lasted even after limited times of being exposed to traumatic events. He was also able to identify the pathways of pathological behaviors that would stay in place for years.

Liddell wrote that one of the main purposes of the farm was to counter Freud's position that neurosis was purely a "human privilege" (Freud, 1939). His ethological approach to studying behaviors consistent with psychopathology in animals brought interested observers from many different fields. He converted many of these professionals to the idea that neurosis could exist across animal species and that there was value in intensely studying what environmental and social factors impacted this pathology, mainly through observational research.

Over the decades that the behavior farm existed, many research papers and presentations were based on the work. Here are just a few examples of the types of findings stressed by the behavior farm research:

- Animals subject to brief mild shocks in the leg led to withdrawal with "neurotic rigidity" that Liddell compared to the psychoanalytic concept of "conversion hysteria".
- Being forcibly isolated and more frequently interacting with researchers carrying out experiments, even if what was involved seemed minor, led to increased nervousness among animals.
- Nervousness in the animals showed a direct relationship with nervousness exhibited by the researchers.
- Each of the individual animals who showed signs of neurosis seemed to have their sources of worry.
- Behaviors reflecting neurosis in the animals were more prominent in those that were more introverted and less social. These were not animals who were forcibly introverted by the researchers who chose to be introverted on their own.

Liddell's work led to his exploring the importance of researchers' interactions with the animals and studying the ways that researcher's behaviors impacted the animals. His focus on the complexity of how all aspects of the animals' environment impacted the animals was what he saw as the best way to identify the comprehensive behavioral structures of experimental neurosis. Focusing on the structures of pathological behaviors, impacted by all aspects of the environment, allowed for identifying the functions of these behaviors. It allowed for the clearest illustration of all behaviors, even those associated with neuroses, had function or purpose. This was the earliest approach to functional behavior analysis, an approach that is still prominent in psychological fields today.

Comparative psychology studies by Liddell showed the value and legitimacy of studying ethology of psychological disorders. This was the concept that psychological disorders existed similarly across different animal species, including humans. His work showed evidence that the behaviors exhibited in neuroses by different animal species were similar as were the factors contributing to those pathological behaviors. Liddell proposed that the behavioral dynamics, for example of anxiety and depressive disorders, were the same across such animal species as humans, pigs, and sheep. His work across many different animal species gave credence to this perspective and provided support for research along this line.

Work from the behavior farm had benefits beyond just research fields. During the Korean War, Liddell worked with the United States military to explore the similarities between neuroses observed on the farm and combat stress in soldiers. He also wrote considerably on parenting styles and what animal studies showed about the more effective styles. His work was widely regarded in positive ways as he presented sheep and goats as ideal examples for understanding effective parenting.

Zoos and Understanding Psychopathology

Following the behavior farm there were many other attempts to study atypical behaviors and psychopathology in zoos. Many of these followed the ethnological work of Liddell, and some researchers even used the term "comparative psychopathology" to describe their work (e.g., Zubin and Hunt). There was a lot of important work in providing material for understanding psychological disorders, although there was no concentrated effort to the degree of Liddell following the behavior farm closing in the 1960s. Ethological and experimental work on psychopathology in zoos continued but in smaller and more diversified ways than in the behavior farm (Chrulew, 2018; Kleinman, 1992).

In the early decades of zoos, there did not seem to be much concern about what living in zoos did to animals. Zoo visitors and employees recognized unusual behaviors that included animals throwing feces at visitors, kicking their cages, and spitting water at visitors and employees. Even with the work being done by Liddell at the behavior farm, zoos for decades did not seem to either recognize or consider the degree to which the zoo environments themselves were causing pathological behaviors. (Meyer-Holzapfel, 1968). Behavioral issues were deemed related to animals functioning differently than in the wild but not necessarily having problems. These behaviors were not identified as any sort of pathology, but when administrators considered them at all, they were seen as differences rather than problems.

It is interesting to consider the history behind zoos and how the lack of concern administrators and other people running zoos had for what zoo environments might be doing to animals. For centuries, there were many versions of zoos, but they were purely the domain of the rich and powerful (Kisling, 2000). One of the earliest examples of a zoo was an Assyrian king who kept captive animals on his property in 1100 B.C. (Lindholm, 2013). Historical records excavated since then have shown many other examples, and up until the late 19th century, almost all were captive animals owned by the rich and/or powerful.

In the 19th century, there were more attempts across the world to build public zoos than there had been before. This was not an easy task and there actually was a lot of resistance to the idea. In the United States, there was an effort starting in 1889 to build a "zoological park" for animals that had been gifted to the United States government (Mann, 1946). Attempts to get funding did not pass, and one of the major problems was that government officials could not say decisively how a zoo would work and even why it was needed.

When a zoological park was finally approved, one of the main arguments that helped was that many of the animals gifted to the government were on the verge of being extinct. It was also successfully argued that any setting used to house these animals would be better than the crowded and overheated setting where they had been housed to that point. There also needed to be money for feeding the animals as the initial sum set aside had already run out.

As zoos developed, allowing the public to see animals was deemed to have a number of benefits. It provided needed financial resources for zoos that charged fees. Having the public visit zoos allowed to education and increased understanding of what animals needed. Appreciation and respect for animals was increased by people seeing how animals lived and functioned. Respecting the need of animals for healthy environments helped to improve conservation efforts and include public approval for this effort.

So, at least in the United States, when public zoos started, there was no concern about what impact the setting had on animals. It was deemed that anything would be better than what the animals had and that zoos would be a way of making sure they were safe and healthy. Keeping these animals away from predators, including humans who hunted them, was seen as worth any environmental difficulties zoos presented.

Behavioral issues, likely reflecting psychopathology, among zoo animals, were noticed, but for many decades, it did not seem there was much concern about them. These would later be deemed evidence of psychopathology directly related to zoo environments, but initially, they were not considered much. Again, one reason is that whatever caused the behaviors was seen as worthwhile because the zoos were keeping animals safe and healthy. It was also the case that the behaviors themselves were often a reason why people visited zoos. Watching a lion or gorilla sit around monitoring their environment for hours might be a little interesting, but lions roaring more frequently than in the jungle or gorillas throwing feces at visitors (both of which can be responses to restricted environments) is what could really get the visitors coming in.

In the first eight decades of their existence, public zoos relied on "hard architecture" where animals were kept in cages. Some aspects of what Sommer (1974) referred to when using this term included concrete boxes, steel bars, and a fixed routine of feeding, watering, and washing. This all distorted the behavior of animals and has been compared to prison and mental hospitals. Over 30 years after initially using that term, Sommer (2008) observed that zoos had undergone considerable changes. He noted that zoos seemed to be the only type of institution with complex architecture that had experienced significant reform.

For many decades, there was little focus on how animals responded to their zoo environments. What changed this sort of thinking was how drastically behaviors changed and mirrored more of the typical behavior seen in the wild, following major changes in how zoos function (Hosey & Skyner, 2007). There was a drastic shift across the zoo community from an emphasis on "hard architecture" to "soft architecture". This shift occurred for many reasons, but one of the main early reasons was to move zoos away from being just attractions and to being more "conservation parks" (Parker, 2021). Although the change was not primarily to address the behaviors exhibited by zoo animals there was a notable change in those behaviors associated with the shift to "soft architecture".

Terry Maple (one of the authors of this book) was instrumental in the movement to modify zoos starting in the 1970s. This work involved making zoos more consistent with the softer design that allowed for more focus on issues important to understanding natural environments. It was also quickly evident that this was also very beneficial for the animals. His work at the Jacksonville Zoo and Gardens Wellness Unit provided multiple studies aimed at quantifying the degree to which certain types of interventions help to promote or maintain species appropriate behaviors and decrease maladaptive behaviors. His work was an important avenue for showing that zoos allow for the opportunity to observe behaviors in many different types of environments, but also the potential for zoos for showing the impact of environmental changes.

As many zoos started changing in the 1970s, it was also clear that they were providing an opportunity to fill an important research gap. Maple and Segura (2015) noted that zoos and zoological parks had the opportunity to become the major, if not the only, facilities where animals can be studied in depth by psychologists. Groupings of animals like chimpanzees and gorillas provide a naturalistic setting, where psychologist can study the mental social and emotional life of these animals. This was noted by these authors to be even more of an important issue than it was in the past, as animal laboratories previously devoted to comparative and behavioral analytic research were being closed. As a result, laboratories as an option to zoos in terms of psychological research are rather limited anyway, because they are becoming less available.

Maple and Segura (2015) reviewed how zoos filled the research gap left when comparative psychology and behavioral analytic laboratories closed over the past decades. They also addressed the important role zoos played in keeping endangered animals safe. Zoos provided an opportunity to study animals in their environments and, as a result, understanding the animals and their environments better. Much like Liddell (1923a), as zoo professionals became more aware of how the animals responded to zoo environments there was more interest in studying why they responded that way. Behavioral issues not evident in the wild were gradually seen as important topics to study in their own right. Whereas earlier these behaviors were often accepted as a necessary even if a negative reality of zoos (i.e. animals showed agitation in response to being in an environment that kept them safer and healthier), it was now recognized that these behaviors were likely related to many different environmental and psychological factors. Zoos were increasingly becoming like the comparative psychopathology laboratories that behavior farms had been years earlier.

What Zoos Provide for Comparative Psychopathology?

Because of the practicality of keeping animals in areas they cannot leave, zoos offer the opportunity to study the impact of restricted spaces. Repetitive behaviors are often associated with restricted spaces, and some of the repetitive behaviors found in zoos include rocking and self-destructive headbanging. Repetitive behaviors in zoos often mimic behaviors that occur in the wild but occur much more often. This includes repetitive pacing that occurs in zoos among bears, who are using the searching behaviors used in the wild but engaging in those behaviors repetitively for no clear purpose. In these behaviors occurring in restricted environments, it is the repetitiveness that differs from behavior in the wild and not the behaviors.

Studying animals in zoos is an important way of studying the impact of restricted environments. Animals in captive environments have shown behavioral abnormalities that include self-mutilation and inappropriate aggression. Behaviors exhibited by animals in more restricted environments resemble symptoms of depression, anxiety disorders, eating disorders, and posttraumatic stress disorders (Bruene et al., 2006). Understanding human psychopathology better by understanding animal psychology follows from how animal models are used to applying understanding of animal physiology to physical illnesses (Keehn, 1982).

Inappropriate aggression and repetitive behaviors are two types of behaviors exhibited often by animals who show problems dealing with restricted environment. Due to the outstanding of social interactions and their extended periods of juvenile dependence, animals like great apes have particular problems dealing with solitary housing and sensory deprivation that had commonly been found in zoos. Studies in zoos showed not only the need to change these environments but also the types of interventions that helped lessen their negative effects. Some interventions found helpful for improving behaviors associated with animals facing difficulties with zoo living include psychopathology, increased efforts to familiarize the individual animals with novel, physical, and social environments, and taking more time and opportunities to re-socialize the animal into the new setting (Brune et al. 2006).

Atypical behaviors most often observed among animals living in zoos include repetitive pacing, self-biting, and consumption of feces (coprophagia). These are the types of behaviors observed at zoos and are the types of behaviors that led to changes in zoos, resulting in the more open and less restricted zoo environments that we see today (Chrulew, 2020). Most relevant among the aspects of zee settings that led to these atypical behaviors were increased enclosure and decreased freedom of movement. These were behaviors seen more often in the early 20th century when there was little effort put into making the environments as close to the natural environments as possible. Once changes were made to make zoos more consistent with natural environments, these behaviors decreased.

Development of the Gorilla Behavior Index (Gold & Maple, 1994) is a good example of a psychological instrument that developed through zoo research. This test is a subjective assessment instrument that consists of behaviorally based average adjectives. It was completed for 298 captive gorillas' hat were over one year of age and was completed over an extended period of time in several zoos. When the data was collected, the results were subjected to common factor analysis, and this resulted in the identification of four main factors, extroverted, dominant, fearful, and understanding. It has been considered a test of animal personality and is one measure used to gauge animal psychopathology.

As a rich source of observational data on psychopathology in animals, zoos provide an important setting for advancing veterinary psychiatry (Binding et al., 2020). This is the field dedicated to not only understanding psychopathology in nonhuman animals but also its treatment. It is a field that has existed for decades but has not formally received much attention. As stated in earlier chapters, there is not much focus to this field and the way it is practiced varies greatly across settings. There is, for example, no text like DSM-5 for veterinary psychiatry and no formal research methods. In addition, there are very few formal training programs in the field.

Ellenberger (1960) listed four characteristics of zoos, including animal behaviors that allow for comparison with human behaviors. When listing these characteristics, the author made direct reference to how the study of animals in zoos could help researchers and practitioners understand better the experiences of individuals living in similar types of confinement, including prisons and hospitals. In this way, studying the impact of confinement on nonhuman animals would help us understand the impact of confinement on human animals. These four characteristics identified by Ellenberger were captivity trauma, nesting, social competition frustration syndrome, and emotional deterioration.

When describing these four characteristics, Ellenberger found that captivity trauma was exemplified by acute agitation and prolonged refusal to eat. Nesting was exhibited by behaviors focused on the establishment of territory, even if there was not very large or meaningful territory to establish. Social competition syndrome was exhibited in the formation of dominance patterns that may or may not have any real benefit in the confined area. Finally, emotional deterioration was expressed as repetitive stereotyped movements with no clear purpose.

These four characteristics seen in zoos were then compared with human responses to confinement, like hospitals and prisons. Behaviors consistent with captivity trauma are exhibited by anger, withdrawal, and severe negativism. Nesting is exhibited by the patient or prisoners establishing the cell or hospital room as a home and fighting over territory; social competition syndrome is exhibited by the interpersonal jealousy and pettiness that often are seen in confined areas; emotional deterioration as exhibited in the form of regressions and catatonic gestures responding to the emotional difficulties experienced in confined settings.

Zoos and Advancing Comparative Psychopathology

When considering what zoos offer for understanding human psychopathology, Ellenberger's work shows how they offer the opportunity to view in detail the impact of major ills of society. They give the opportunity to study how human psychopathology is impacted negatively by the lack of what society considers necessities. Like zoos for nonhuman animals, prisons and hospitals have real benefits for human society. Zoos keep animals confined, but they allow for the opportunity for humans, who undoubtedly have more control over what happens to these animals' environments to better these animals. They allow humans to not only appreciate animals and connect with them but also see directly how the animals rely on what the natural world provides. Although they have benefits they also require the loss of freedom and the presence of confinement.

Similarly, hospitals and prisons provide necessities for human society. They are needed to keep all humans healthy and safe. It could be argued that they exist as much for the benefit of society than just for the individual (Goldman, 2020). As a result, they often have negative consequences for the individual even if they are also providing positives for the individual (e.g., prisoners could be said to be benefiting from learning the consequences of their actions) and society. These negatives relate primarily to the restrictions and confinement these settings require. In this context, zoos as a part of comparative psychopathology research, would offer the opportunity not only to further understand specific factors that contribute to psychopathology but also to understand what happens when environmental factors that people often associate with living positive lives or nonexistent or are taken away.

Looking at the role that zoos can play in the totality of comparative psychopathology allows for consideration of one way this approach is different from other approaches to understanding psychopathology. Since the beginning of psychology as a separate field, one criticism has been its reliance on research and practice involving humans at the higher levels of human society. Freud and Jung developed psychoanalysis with patients from the upper income levels of society. Psychotherapy practitioners (e.g., Anna Freud, Otto Rank, Eric Reich) also based their theories and therapy approaches on working with patients who had higher incomes and higher levels of education. The same is true of authors and practitioners prominent in developing other major schools of psychotherapy theories (e.g., cognitive-behavior therapy and humanistic therapy).

Psychology research has also suffered from the limitation of relying too heavily on humans from the upper levels of society (Appio et al., 2013; Liddell, 2005; Sunar, 1978). This is made most prominent in the criticism that psychology research is much too slanted in its reliance on college and university students. This criticism also applies to how human psychology research has relied too heavily on groups which yield disproportionate power in Western society (healthy white males being the most prominent here). This is an issue that psychology has addressed in recent decades, but it continues to be a major concern.

In its reliance on individuals who belong to groups that have more ready access to what society deems important (e.g.,, money, political power, voices that are readily heard), psychology has clearly leaned too much in recognizing how psychological functioning is impacted by having enough (Leeder, 1996). Even understanding major psychological disorders like schizophrenia can be slanted if that understanding is based on impaired individuals who are verbal and have access to even modest incomes and freedom. This leads to psychological theories based on an understanding of what having "enough" resources means and how it impacts functioning (Williams, 2020).

It could be argued, based on its reliance on individuals who have "enough" of what society requires, that psychology has too often relied on a "top-down" approach to understanding psychopathology. It starts with looking at how psychopathology as it develops from individuals who are at the "top" in terms of what society offers. Psychopathology is understood then as it relates to functioning for individuals who otherwise have what their society requires (even if it is only in modest amount). Once that is addressed, individuals with less (e.g. less income, less freedom, less verbal ability, less independence) are focused on to the degree that resources (e.g. research money, faculty time) allow. Psychology then becomes limited in terms of what it fully offers in understanding what it means for people to have less than what is needed for "normal" functioning in society. Describing the study of psychopathology as "abnormal" psychology is limited in that it only addresses deviation from what people need for psychological functioning but does not fully incorporate the impact of lacking other resources.

Comparative psychopathology, in contrast, can be seen as an approach that takes a "down-top" approach when considering the impact of having less than what society requires. Relying on research on zoos allows for understanding the psychological impact of less freedom than others in society. This builds on comparative psychopathology's emphasis, much more than other approaches, of research relying on species that do not emphasize verbal language. It is also relying on research for species that do not have the same level of cognitive functioning consistent with "average" human intellectual functioning. This lack of cognitive abilities expected of humans would not interfere with animal functioning but is consistent with impaired human functioning.

Comparative psychopathology, as a result of it incorporating variables associated with lower functioning in humans, allows for a truly comprehensive way of understanding the human experience. Looking at what factors impact psychopathology when individuals function with verbal language abilities or other cognitive abilities allows for a stronger understanding of the impact of these situations than the more "top-down" approaches. When it comes to zoos making up a large part of comparative psychopathology research, this allows for incorporating an understanding of what living in restricted environments means for psychological functioning. Individuals living without those things deemed important for human society become central to comparative psychopathology and not just ancillary based on the "leftovers" of what researchers and theorists have available.

Looking at comparative psychopathology this way, it is an approach to understanding a major psychology area that incorporates up front experiences of those living without resources deemed by society to be important. Experiences consistent with humans living in prisons, nursing homes, hospitals, group homes and other restricted environments is essential. It emphasizes research of experiences consistent with those faced by humans with intellectual, social and communication impairments. This is something that has been missing from other approaches to psychopathology (Nezu & Nezu, 1994; Witwer et al., 2022). Experiences consistent with those of people with autism, intellectual disability, and communication disorders make a larger part of comparative psychopathology's focus than is the case with other approaches to understanding psychopathology.

Zoos as research hubs in comparative psychopathology allows for intensive study of individuals experiencing lack of resources and independence. This allows for studying psychological constructs similar to humans living in other restricted environments. It also emphasizes studying experiences consistent with humans suffering the most restrictive factor of all, poverty. Nonhuman animals living in zoos face severe restrictions on what they can do, very limited control over their environment and lack of resources deemed important for human societies. These are the same issues faced by individual living in poverty (Reiman & Leighton, 2020). Studying psychopathology as it exists in zoos allows for studying the impact of major factors also important in lives of humans suffering poverty.

Poverty as a major variable has been minimized in many approaches to understanding psychopathology and its treatment (Acosta et al., 1982). There has not been a major approach to understanding psychopathology that has incorporated the psychological impact of poverty prominently. Powerlessness and lack of resources also have not stood out at the very base of how schools of thought understand psychopathology and human experiences. When poverty, powerlessness and lack of resources have been part of psychological schools of thought, this has typically been as a modifier to approaches and theories already in place. Examples include disability studies (Goodley, 2021), poverty studies (Frankenhuis & Nettle, 2020), integrative psychotherapy theory (Williams Kapten, 2020), and recognition theory (Gilmartin et al., 2023). Comparative psychopathology provides a new path that incorporates the role of powerless, lack of resources found important in human society and different abilities into a comprehensive psychological approach.

References

Acosta, F. X., Yamamoto, J., Evans, L. A., Acosta, F. X., Yamamoto, J., Evans, L. A., & Wilcox, S. A. (1982). *Effective Psychotherapy for Low-Income and Minority Patients* (pp. 1–29). Springer US.

Appio, L., Chambers, D. A., & Mao, S. (2013). Listening to the voices of the poor and disrupting the silence about class issues in psychotherapy. *Journal of Clinical Psychology*, *69*(2), 152–161.

Ayala, A. J., Haas, L. K., Williams, B. M., Fink, S. S., Yabsley, M. J., & Hernandez, S. M. (2022). Risky business in Georgia's wild birds: contact rates between wild birds and backyard chickens is influenced by supplemental feed. *Epidemiology & Infection, 150.*

Binding, S., Farmer, H., Krusin, L., & Cronin, K. (2020). Status of animal welfare research in zoos and aquariums: Where are we, where to next?. *Journal of Zoo and Aquarium Research, 8*(3), 166–174.

Block, J. D. (1963). In memoriam: Howard S. Liddell, Ph.D. 1895–1962. *Psychosomatic Medicine, 25*, 1–2.

Broadhurst, P. L. (1960). Abnormal animal behaviour. In: H. J. Eysenck (Ed.), *Handbook of Abnormal Psychology: An Experimental Approach* (pp. 726–763). London: Pitman Medical Publishing Ltd.

Bruene, M., Brüne-Cohrs, U., McGrew, W. C., & Preuschoft, S. (2006). Psychopathology in great apes: Concepts, treatment options and possible homologies to human psychiatric disorders. *Neuroscience & Biobehavioral Reviews, 30*(8), 1246–1259.

Chrulew, M. (2018). Living, biting monitors, a morose howler and other infamous animals: Animal biographies in ethology and zoo biology. *Animal Biography: Re-Framing Animal Lives*, 19–40.

Chrulew, M. (2020). Abnormal animals. *New Literary History, 51*(4), 729–750.

Clark, R. A. (1955). Jung and Freud: A chapter in psychoanalytic history. *American Journal of Psychotherapy, 9*(4), 605–611.

Clay, A. S., & Visseren-Hamakers, I. J. (2022). Individuals matter: Dilemmas and solutions in conservation and animal welfare practices in zoos. *Animals, 12*(3), 398.

Ellenberger, H. F. (1960). Zoological Garden and Mental Hospital. *Canadian Psychiatric Association Journal, 5*(3),136–149. doi:10.1177/070674376000500302

Fernandez, E. J., & Martin, A. L. (2021). Animal training, environmental enrichment, and animal welfare: A history of behavior analysis in zoos. *Journal of Zoological and Botanical Gardens, 2*(4), 531–543.

Frankenhuis, W. E., & Nettle, D. (2020). The strengths of people in poverty. *Current Directions in Psychological Science, 29*(1), 16–21.

Freud, S. (1939) *Moses and Monotheism.* New York: Vintage Books.

Gamble, A., Olarte-Castillo, X. A., & Whittaker, G. R. (2023). Backyard zoonoses: The roles of companion animals and peri-domestic wildlife. *Science Translational Medicine, 15*(718), eadj0037.

Gilmartin, D., McElvaney, R., & Corbally, M. (2023). "Talk to me like I'ma human" An interpretative phenomenological analysis of the psychotherapy experiences of young people in foster care in Ireland. *Counselling Psychology Quarterly, 36*(1), 66–88.

Gold, K.C., & Maple, T.L. (1994). Personality assessment in the gorilla and its utility as a management tool. *Zoo Biology,13*, 509–522.

Goldman, E. (2020). *Prisons: A social crime and failure* (Vol. 1). Library of Alexandria.

Goodley, D. (2021). Disability studies and human encounters. *Indian Journal of Critical Disability Studies, 1*(1), 12–21.

Greenwell, P. J., Riley, L. M., Lemos de Figueiredo, R., Brereton, J. E., Mooney, A., & Rose, P. E. (2023). The societal value of the modern zoo: A commentary on how zoos can positively impact on human populations locally and globally. *Journal of Zoological and Botanical Gardens, 4*(1), 53–69.

Hopper, Lydia M. (2017). Cognitive research in zoos. *Current Opinion in Behavioral Sciences* 16, 100–110.

Hosey, G. R., & Skyner, L. J. (2007). Self-injurious behavior in zoo primates. *International Journal of Primatology*, *28*, 1431–1437.

Janmaat, K. R. (2019). What animals do not do or fail to find: A novel observational approach for studying cognition in the wild. *Evolutionary Anthropology: Issues, News, and Reviews*, *28*(6), 303–320.

Keehn, J. D. (1982). Psychopathology in animals. *New Zealand Psychologist*.

Kirk, R. G., & Ramsden, E. (2018). Working across species down on the farm: Howard S. Liddell and the development of comparative psychopathology, c. 1923–1962. *History and Philosophy of the Life Sciences*, *40*, 1–29.

Kisling, V. N. (Ed.). (2000). *Zoo and aquarium history: Ancient animal collections to zoological gardens*. CRC press.

Kleiman, D. G. (1992). Behavior research in zoos: Past, present, and future. *Zoo Biology*, *11*(5), 301–312.

Kögler, J., Pacheco, I. B., & Dierkes, P. W. (2020). Evaluating the quantitative and qualitative contribution of zoos and aquaria to peer-reviewed science. *Journal of zoo and Aquarium Research*, *8*(2), 124–132.

Kummrow, M. S., & Brüne, M. (2018). Psychopathologies in captive nonhuman primates and approaches to diagnosis and treatment. *Journal of Zoo and Wildlife Medicine*, *49*(2), 259–271.

Learmonth, M. J. (2020). Human–animal interactions in zoos: What can compassionate conservation, conservation welfare and duty of care tell us about the ethics of interacting, and avoiding unintended consequences? *Animals*, *10*(11), 2037.

Leeder, E. (1996). Speaking rich people's words: Implications of a feminist class analysis of psychotherapy. *Women & Therapy*, *18*(3–4), 45–57.

Liddell, H. S. (1923a). Some methods for investigating the effect of thyroidectomy on the neuro-muscular mechanism of sheep. *Quarterly Journal of Experimental Physiology*, *13*, 191–197.

Liddell, H. S. (1923b). The possible influence of fatigue on the reaction time of thyroidectomized sheep. *Proceedings of the Society for Experimental Biology and Medicine*, *21*(2), 126–127.

Liddell, H. S. (1925a). The growth of the head in thyroidectomized sheep. *The Anatomical Record*, *30*(5), 327–332.

Liddell, H. S. (1925b). The relation between maze learning and spontaneous activity in the sheep. *Journal of Comparative Psychology*, *5*(6), 475.

Liddell, H. S. (1926). The effect of thyroidectomy on some unconditioned responses of the sheep and goat. *American Journal of Physiology-Legacy Content*, *75*(3), 579–590.

Liddell, H. S. (1927). Higher nervous activity in the thyroidectomised sheep and goat. *Quarterly Journal of Experimental Physiology: Translation and Integration*, *17*(1), 41–51.

Liddell, H. S. (1954). Conditioning and emotions. *Scientific American*, *190*(1), 48–57.

Liddell, L. (2005). Psychotherapy, classism, and the poor: Conspicuous by their absence. *American Psychologist*, *60*(7), 687–696. https://doi.org/10.1037/0003-066X.60.7.687

Lindholm, J. (2013). Zoo history. In: M. D. Irwin, J. B. Stoner, & A. M. Cobaugh, (Eds.), *Zookeeping: An Introduction to the Science and Technology* (pp. 31–42).

Mann, W. (1946). A brief history of the zoo. *The Scientific Monthly*, *63*(5), 350–358.

Maple, T. L., & Segura, V. D. (2015). Advancing behavior analysis in zoos and aquariums. *The Behavior Analyst*, *38*, 77–91.

Meyer-Holzapfel, M. (1968). Abnormal behavior in zoo animals. In: M. Fox (Ed.), *Abnormal Behavior in Animals* (pp. 476–503). Philadelphia, PA: W.B. Saunders Co.

Miranda, R., Escribano, N., Casas, M., Pino-del-Carpio, A., & Villarroya, A. (2023). The role of zoos and aquariums in a changing world. *Annual Review of Animal Biosciences, 11,* 287–306.

Nezu, C. M., & Nezu, A. M. (1994). Outpatient psychotherapy for adults with mental retardation and concomitant psychopathology: Research and clinical imperatives. *Journal of Consulting and Clinical Psychology, 62*(1), 34.

Parker, M. (2021). The genealogy of the zoo: Collection, park and carnival. *Organization, 28*(4), 604–620.

Reiman, J., & Leighton, P. (2020). *The rich get richer and the poor get prison: Thinking critically about class and criminal justice.* Routledge.

Schubart, W. (1989). The patient in the analyst's consulting room-the first consultation as a psychoanalytic encounter. *The International Journal of Psycho-Analysis, 70,* 423.

Sommer, R. (1974). *Tight Spaces: Hardarchitecture and How to Humanize It.* Englewood Cliffs, NJ: Prentice-Hall.

Sommer, R. (2008). Development of the zoological garden and mental hospital. *American Journal of Orthopsychiatry, 78,* 378–382.

Spooner, S. L., Walker, S. L., Dowell, S., & Moss, A. (2023). The value of zoos for species and society: The need for a new model. *Biological Conservation, 279,* 109925.

Sunar, D.G. (1978). Stereotypes of the powerless: A social psychological analysis. *Psychological Reports, 43*(2), 511–528.

Williams Kapten, S. (2020). Power, powerlessness, and the parallel process. *Journal of Psychotherapy Integration, 30*(1), 147–154. https://doi.org/10.1037/int0000168

Williams, M. T. (2020). Psychology cannot afford to ignore the many harms caused by microaggressions. *Perspectives on Psychological Science, 15*(1), 38–43.

Witwer, A. N., Rosencrans, M. E., Held, M. K., Cobranchi, C., Crane, J., Chapman, R., Havercamp, S. M., & The Ohio State University Nisonger RRTC on Health and Function. (2022). Psychotherapy treatment outcome research in adults with ID: Where do we go from here? *Clinical Psychology: Science and Practice.* Advance online publication. https://doi.org/10.1037/cps0000053

9 Aggression and Comparative Psychopathology

Introduction

In discussing comparative psychopathology, we have looked at how this approach can help better understand psychological constructs associated with more prevalent psychological disorders. In the final two chapters of this book, we will look at the role comparative psychopathology can serve in understanding two of the more prominent behavioral categories: aggression and deprivation-induced pathologies. These are not behavioral categories associated with any specific disorder but serve a major role in multiple psychological disorders.

It could easily be argued that aggression is one of the most, if not the most, impactful of all behavioral categories studied by psychology. Violence, murder, property damage, threats, intimate partner abuse, and assaults cause unbearable pain and suffering to millions across the world. If the world holds out hope that psychology can help explain and contain any behavioral pathologies, violence, and aggression likely top the list. Comparative psychopathology offers help in this process by providing additional ways of understanding aggression.

Aggression and Psychological Disorders

Aggressive behaviors are not associated with any one psychological disorder but are associated with several different formal psychological disorders (Haller, 2022; Mos & Olivier, 1991; Pompili et al., 2017). These disorders include bipolar disorder, borderline personality disorder, mood disorders, posttraumatic stress disorder, conduct disorder, and impulse control disorder (Coccaro & Lee, 2020). It is interesting that aggression is a possible symptom of each diagnosis but only one, Intermittent Explosive Disorder, is identified as primarily a diagnosis of pathological physical aggression.

Psychology recognizes that defensive aggression (e.g., aggression to safeguard the safety of oneself and/or one's family) is a normal behavior pattern

DOI: 10.4324/9781003408918-10

that occurs throughout human development. What becomes interesting when studying psychopathology is the issue of pathological aggression. It is not easy to define when aggression becomes pathological (i.e., goes beyond that which is necessary for defensive aggression), but it does represent a major area of concern when studying psychological disorders.

Aggression in psychological disorders is a legitimate area of concern as it represents the behavioral component most dangerous to others when someone has a psychological disorder. Problems with mood, comprehension, focus, and reality testing can cause problems for others, but it is the aggressive behaviors that present consistent danger. This area of concern has been so evident that it has been problematic. People with psychological disorders are often stereotyped as being dangerous even though dangerous physical aggression is not more prevalent among this population than other populations (Hiday, 1995; Varshney et al., 2015). There are psychological disorders with aggression as a behavioral symptom, but as a whole, people with psychological disorders are not more physically aggressive.

For years, pathological aggression was split into two primary categories: impulsive and premediated aggression (Coccaro, 2012), also known as reactive and proactive aggression (Pisano & Masi, 2020). Impulsive aggression is associated with emotional reactivity and rule-breaking, while premeditated aggression is associated with the expectation of a reward or achieving a goal. Impulsive aggression is an emotionally charged act resulting from minimal provocation, while premeditated aggression is a planned and conscious act not attached to any particular emotional state (Babcock et al., 2014). Impulsive aggression is considered to be the primary type of aggression associated with Impulse Control Disorder. Premeditated aggression is considered to be primarily associated with Antisocial Personality Disorder, although there is research suggesting that this disorder is more associated with impulsive aggression (Azevedo et al., 2020).

There are a number of differences between the two types of pathological aggression, impulsive and premeditated, among humans (Barratt et al., 1999). Impulsive aggression is more often associated with guilt and remorse. Premediated occurs for increased dominance and social gain. Individuals who engage in premediated aggression are more likely to re-offend than those involved with impulsive aggression. Impulsive aggression responds better to anger management training, focused on developing better skills for handling anger, while premeditated aggression responds better to cognitive restructuring, focused on altering how the individual views the world and social relationships.

Although the impulsive/premediated dichotomy has been a useful one for understanding human aggression it has been legitimately criticized as being too simplistic. Its focus on describing essentially two clearly different types of aggression often minimizes how much different types of aggressive acts have in common. It also fails to account for aggression that has multiple motives (Bushman & Anderson, 2001).

Critics of the impulsive/premeditated dichotomy approach to understanding human aggression have offered an alternative, called a "knowledge structure" approach (Garofalo et al., 2021; Huesmann, 1998). In this approach to understanding aggression, individuals develop sets of interrelated information stored in memory that, over time, become activated by the same type of situations. These sets of interrelated information get activated together so often that they become strongly linked and over time are automatically activated by similar situations. Their interconnectedness is strengthened by how early on and how frequently they are learned together.

In the case of aggression, interconnected information is learned about how to deal with situations where the individual perceives a threat. This could be a challenge to their resources or to their survival. This could also be situations that come to be associated with the affective state, with its cognitive and physiological components, that is often called "anger". Introduction of this affective state could determine whether the person acts immediately based on knowledge structures or whether additional calculation is required (hereby including a step that crosses over between the impulsive and premeditated models). Either way, the knowledge structures either immediately or eventually lead the individual to act in learned ways to handle the situations that the individual has interpreted as a "threat," and that has triggered the emotional state the individual has named "anger."

This knowledge structure approach to understanding aggression allows for a comparative discussion of aggression involving both human and nonhuman animals. It presents a view of aggression that crosses over the main constructs for understanding aggression across virtually all species. It presents aggression as a learned pattern of behavior and, as such, implicates (as is done when discussing learning processes) the role of rewards and punishments. Aggression, as we will see, is strongly influenced by the degree to which the individual finds rewards in the aggressive behaviors. This model also views aggression as specifically a matter of social learning, influenced not just by the interpersonal situation but also by social standings and social hierarchies. It also emphasizes aggression as a behavioral pattern often triggered by physiological and cognitive experiences that humans associate with the affective state called "anger". Each of these is an important psychological construct in the discussion of aggression, regardless of the animal species involved.

Aggression and the Animal World

Aggression is a one social behavior that exists across all animal species. It is an essential behavior used for securing resources necessary for survival and for protecting self and family (Albert et al., 1993; Jager et al., 2020;

Lischinsky & Lin, 2020; Range & Marshall-Pescini, 2022; Van Heukelum et al., 2021). It is considered a highly functional type of social behavior used to gain and maintain important resources. These resources including territory, food, mates, and water. If it were not for aggressive behaviors to a certain degree, animals (including humans) would starve, die of thirst, have no place to live, and/or be without the means to reproduce. This shows aggression to have an essential place in ensuring survival for all animal species.

It is clear aggression holds an essential place throughout the animal world. Animals would quickly lose their homes and access to food and water if they did not fight off rivals. They would get killed and eaten quickly if they did not fight off predators (and predators would die off quickly if they were not aggressive toward prey). Humans would be overrun, dominated, and likely killed if they did not fight off opponents for needed resources (Blanchard & Blanchard, 2003). They also would be subject to loss of freedom and dominance by others if they did not fight opponents. Humans would also be killed quickly if they did not fight off predators (showing the importance not only of inter-species aggression but also intra-species aggression).

Physical aggression holds its essential place not just because it directly leads to obtaining or keeping needed resources (e.g. food, shelter, mates). It is primarily because physical aggression is how members of a species show dominance over others. Dominance in social hierarchies is the reason members have more access to resources and is the most obvious reason why aggression, used to obtain and maintain dominance, is so essential (Resta et al., 2023). Aggression is used to obtain dominance and then, once dominance is obtained, other behaviors (e.g. punishment, threats) are used to maintain it (Tibbetts et al., 2022).

Knowledge plays an important role in aggression, not only in terms of understanding what behaviors work but also what information is needed. Research shows that animals who analyze more social information are often better able to optimize who they challenge for dominance (Hobson, 2020). Strategies used to pick fights and engage in aggression for social dominance depend strongly on the social information available. There are various theories about how social information is used and the most parsimonious is that decisions about aggression involve a simple summation of relevant factors without a detailed analysis of relative abilities (Elwood & Arnott, 2012). Animals do not necessarily need to decide that they are the most competent fighters if they can effectively analyze whether important factors make a fight beneficial. Important information includes knowing how the hierarchies work and what is expected in the social hierarchies (Hobson et al., 2021; Shizuka & McDonald, 2015).

Since learning models play a large role in understanding pathological aggression, as we will discuss soon, it is useful to look at how learning and aggression operate in the nonhuman animal world. Animals (dogs, for example) create a social hierarchy within their species and this hierarchy determines who is dominant within the social group and will be allowed access to needed resources (food, shelter, etc.) without a fight (Corsetti et al., 2021; Jacobs et al., 2003; Riemer et al., 2021; Van den Berg et al., 2008). Here, an interesting point is that reaching the higher points on the hierarchy does not mean the individual animal will fight and win, but reaching the higher levels means the animal will not have to fight (they communicate to lower animals that it is not worth fighting them because they will likely lose). Animals at the top tend to stay on top because they have fought and won but do not need to keep fighting in order to maintain dominance (Natarajan & Caramaschi, 2010).

Notice how these fits in with the social competition theory presented in the depression chapter. Behaviors consistent with depression occur because animals who learn they are lower on the dominance hierarchy stay away from fighting because they realize that fighting will likely lead to a loss and very possibly serious danger or even death. They may fight at times to see if their hierarchy status is still accurate but they exhibit behaviors consistent with defeat is not something they have to do constantly. Material on how aggression works to help animals reach and keep higher levels on the dominance hierarchy works in the other direction. Animals fight to reach higher points on the hierarchy but one benefit of the hierarchy model (which is learned by all animals in a species) is that reaching higher levels signals dominance and animals do not have to fight constantly to maintain dominance.

Looking at the methods by which dominance is maintained without constant aggression provides insight into different types of behaviors associated with aggression. Ritualized behaviors are what help communicate dominance and the likelihood of aggression. Behaviors used in a ritualized way to communicate the upcoming possibility of aggression are called "threat displays." This allows animals to show their relative size and likely skills for a physical conflict (Huntingford & Turner, 1987). In nonhuman animals, this is exhibited through physical actions, while with humans, it is also done by words. This is where some connection exists with what humans' call "verbal aggression" (i.e. use of words to engage in conflict as an alternative to engaging in physical conflict). Aggressive behaviors are learned and maintained most through a fixed-ration or fixed-interval schedule of reinforcement (May & Kennedy, 2009; Portegal, 1979; Thompson, 1961; Thompson, 1966). Physical conflicts may have to occur on a regular basis to maintain dominance, but fighting is not necessarily used on a constant-reinforcement basis (again indicating that dominance is not maintain by fighting in every potential conflict).

Pathological Aggression

Although aggression is considered a necessity it can become pathological. This is when it goes over what is needed for survival (Harat et al., 2015; Sluyter, Takahashi & Maxson, 2014; Wagel et al., 2022). In human societies aggression becoming pathological is often associated with what is meant by the term "violent" (Onyike & Lyketsos, 2011). When physical aggression crosses over from what is considered necessary into behavior humans call "violent" then this enters into the realm of pathological aggression. Consideration of aggression that can be pathological and reflective of atypical psychological development, rather than violent people being "bad" in a moral sense, has its roots early in psychotherapy discourse. Sigmund Freud made frequent reference to aggressive impulses but one of the earliest psychologists to study pathological aggression and its similarity to, but deviation from, typical human development was hist daughter, Anna Freud (Freud, 1947).

When studying aggression in animals living in the wild, it is often difficult to define when aggression becomes pathological. This is because aggression is so often needed out in the wild that it is difficult to distinguish when it becomes more than what is necessary. It is difficult to define when aggression becomes excessive out in the wild because it is difficult to determine there when aggression stops being a necessary means of survival (Eibl-Eibesfeldt, 1977). However, since the 1990s there have been more studies than before of pathological and excessive aggression in nonhuman animals (Covington III et al., 2019). These include studies of raids on neighboring troops by chimpanzees, impulsive and excessive attacks by rodents, and atypical violence exhibited by mice.

Research on pathological aggression in nonhuman animals identify one major contributing factor common throughout most studies, physical aggression becomes pathological because the behavior itself becomes rewarding. Pathological aggression is associated with physical aggression, and its association with winning and dominance, because the individual finds it rewarding beyond what is needed for survival. Studies on animals exhibiting deviant violence showed that these animals would seek out opportunities to attack, even if there was not obvious benefit to the conflict. This pattern of aggressive behaviors itself becoming rewarding could be due to some sort of brain injury, deviant neurological pathways or operant conditioning (Bandura et al., 1963; Lee et al. 2008; Loew, 1967). Human pathological aggression has similar causes (Haller & Kruk, 2006): brain dysfunction, physiological hypoarousal that limits the emotional barriers that hinder violence (like in antisocial personality disorder) and hyperarousal that leads to irritability and angry outbursts (present in psychological disorders like Intermittent Explosive Disorder and clinical depression). Hyperarousal, as described here, is associated with a learning process involving operant conditioning, where fighting becomes a reward for reasons other than overt reasons.

Pathological aggression has been compared to a sort of "addiction" in that the individual finds aggressiveness rewarding outside of any clear external reinforcement (Kuik, 2022). There is a positive reward feeling following the attack that is evident from neurological evidence, even if there is no clear social benefit to the aggression. This proneness for finding aggressive behaviors reinforced continued in animals even after a period of forced abstinence (Golden et al., 2017). There is evidence from mice studies of a genetic predisposition that leads to individuals being more prone to finding aggression itself reinforcing after a period of time when the behavior is reinforced by some other reinforcer on a fixed schedule (Fish et al., 2002). This may be the same type of genetic predisposition that makes individuals prone to impulsivity (Coppens et al., 2014; Miczek et al., 2007; Van Heukelum et al., 2021).

From a neurological perspective, aggression overlaps with the same neural networks associated with adaptive social behaviors, like play, sex, parenting and bonding (Kohl et al., 2017; Li & Dulac, 2018). Dopamine levels increase and signal neurologically that winning a confrontation is a desired outcome. As a rewarded experience, fighting and winning fights increases dopamine level the same way as other rewarded behaviors (Couppis & Kennedy, 2008). Winning a confrontation is a positive experience and can lead to aggression becoming a rewarded behavior. When fighting becomes pathological it is because winning the conflict, and the physiological and cognitive response to winning, becomes a reward beyond just what social benefit it provides.

Physical aggression exists in animal species to help individuals have access to resources. Dominance is key in the purpose to why aggression is exists and why it is used. This is part of the natural course by which non-pathological aggression develops. When aggression becomes pathological it is most often because the aggressive behaviors itself become rewarding, separate from any over benefit to the aggression. Individuals with defiant levels of anger do so because they obtain rewards from the aggressive behaviors themselves. As covered so far, this could be because of deviant neurological pathways or because of deviant learning. Different schedules of reinforcement can lead to the individual being reinforced for aggressive beyond the reinforcement provided by the individual's environment.

This view of aggression fits in with the knowledge structure view of pathological aggression discussed earlier. Physical aggression is learned as a behavioral pattern used in situations where the individual feels threatened, perceives an opportunity to obtain needed resources or experiences a physiological and cognitive responses that humans describe with the affective word "anger". This is the typical way aggression develops and in pathological aggression the triggers for aggression go beyond what is obvious. Individuals prone to pathological aggression have another reason for they the knowledge structure associated with aggression is triggered, they perceive the opportunity for a reward response. They become more sensitive to responding to any situation that shows the potential for experiencing the positive physiological and cognitive responses associated with being aggressive. Individuals learn that aggression will results in the rewarding experiences beyond what others observing the situations perceive.

Aggressive behaviors, especially those associated with psychopathology, often appear inconsistent with what is observed in environmental factors. Severity of aggressive behavior is often not related directly to the severity of overt context (Berkowitz, 1983). When individual animals are described as showing pathological aggression they are often described as acting out of sync with what the obvious context shows. They may be described as seeming more sensitive to what is happening than others who do not show pathological aggression. It is here that we see the important role that sensitivity to environmental triggers plays in pathological aggression. Individuals showing pathological aggression may be more sensitive to others related to what they respond to in the environment. This could be increased sensitivity either to evidence of danger in the environment or sensitivity to what aspects of the environment signal likelihood of reinforcement.

Discussing sensitivity and its role in pathological aggression is important here because decreasing sensitivity to environmental stimuli is a major part of animal domestication. Domestication is seen primarily as a process by which animals are taught to have less sensitivity to environmental triggers (Price, 1999). Domesticated animals are typically expected to have aggression levels that are much lower than animals in the wild. If a domesticated animal showed the same level of physical aggression shown by an animal in the wild that aggression would certainly be deemed pathological. What triggers aggressive responses out in the wild (noises, strangers, environmental changes) needs to be reduced in terms of their impact on triggering aggressive behaviors through domestication.

Given the similar constructs between domestication and addressing pathological aggression (i.e. their importance on reducing sensitivity to environmental stimuli) it is useful to look at what behavioral processes most help in animal domestication. What has changed most in recent years with the process of animal domestication is a focus on rewarding what behaviors are sought rather than punishing the behaviors that are not sought (Greenebaum, 2010; Prunier et al., 2020). Animals are rewarded for showing behaviors that exhibit control over how they respond to environmental stimuli rather than punished for exhibiting any behavior in response to stimuli. This focus on "learning what TO DO and not WHAT NOT TO DO" has shown strong effectiveness in improving attempts at animal domestication. It has also been praised through the animal behavior literature as it focuses on the animal's "otherness" (e.g. treating a dog as a dog rather than trying to make it an altogether different type of animal (Wlodarczyk, 2017).

It is useful consider that the approaches to psychological interventions focused on helping individuals learn new ways of coping (i.e. learning alternative ways of responding) and also emphasizing the individual being treated as an individual is consistent with what in psychotherapy has come to be known as the "positive psychology" movement (Prinzing, 2021). This approach has been effective for human settings by helping decrease bullying (Arslan et al., 2021; García-Vázquez et al., 2020), decreasing cyber-bullying (Agbaria, 2021), prevent aggressive behaviors in children (Owens & Waters, 2020) and decrease physical discipline used by parents (Cui & Lan, 2020).

Other Factors Impacting Aggression

Research on human and nonhuman animals shows that pathological aggression most often starts in the earlier stages of development and in the primary social networks. How families and other caregivers reinforce aggression impacts a great deal on whether an individual growing up in that family develops pathological aggression. Human psychology research shows that pathological aggression is often learned and that living in an uncivil family setting can lead to aggressive behaviors among human adolescents at school and activities and also adults in the workplace (Bai et al., 2020). Aggressive behaviors associated with family incivility include physical aggression (e.g. punching) and non-physical aggression (e.g. cyberbullying). This type of human aggression is consistent with the theory that pathological aggression is learned as a way to deal with situations that would not trigger aggression for most individuals.

Comparative psychology research (summarized in Takahashi, 2021) shows three types of social stressors strongly related to aggression. Social instigation involves interactions with a rival for needed resources (or resources that the individual perceives as needed). Social aggression itself is also a factor. Individuals who win conflicts tend to repeat the same types of aggression that helped them win, even if other reinforcers for the behaviors are not apparent. Social isolation also tends to prompt and reinforce aggression. This often depends on the stage of development at which the individual started experiencing social isolation.

What these three categories of social stressors show are the types of settings that are most prone to reinforce aggression. In human environments, an example of social instigation would be fights at school or playground. These are settings where aggression may be reinforced and have a stronger impact given they are associated with early stages of development (i.e. childhood). Children spending time in settings where social instigations occur are reinforced for aggression when they "win" the fights. This is an example of social aggression and its rewarding potential. Children seek social approval and winning fights, or at least looking like the individual is winning fights, can provide that social approval. Human children who are left alone develop less socially desirable skills and often come to rely on more basic and instinctual ways of dealing with anger and desire for dominance. This is one example of how social isolation contributes to a reliance on human aggression.

Similarly, these same three major social stressors are important for understanding high levels of aggression, and possibly pathological aggression, in nonhuman animals. Animals who are around other animals looking to fight face frequent social instigation and come to rely heavily on fighting behaviors. When animals are good at fighting and show they can win fights, their social aggression is reinforced and tends to occur more often. Animals who are not socialized at all, by remaining isolated during early stages of development, tend to rely on more basic and instinctual behaviors for handling any difficulties. This is why social isolated animals tend to rely more often than others on aggressive behaviors, even beyond the time their aggressive behaviors are reinforced overtly by social acceptance.

Social isolation seems to have a particularly strong impact on human aggression. Isolation from others starting at an early age development has shown more promise for understanding pathological aggression than any other factor in psychological and neurobiology studies (Miczek et al., 2013). Research about teenage human aggression and its rise during the COVID-19 pandemic showed evidence that lack of physical contact may have been a major contributing factor (Field, 2021). This was consistent with animal research showing monkey species who receive more physical touch as adolescents tend to be less aggressive than those that receive less (Reite et al., 1978; Suomi, 2005) It is not only physical contact from others that contributes to aggression but any reinforcers social contact brings. Mice studies have shown that withholding of any social reinforcement can lead to aggression caused by frustration (de Almeida & Miczek, 2002).

Aggression relates to attempts at achieving dominance. Dominance is exhibited and defined different ways throughout the animal world. In the human animal world attempts at dominance can be defined as attempts at achieving significance (Resta et al., 2023). Pathological aggression in this way, for humans, can be seen as a result of individuals seeking dominance by being called and treated by others in ways, they define as being seen as "significant." Being seen as a "significant" individual in one's social network has a strong impact on reinforcing behaviors leading to that term being used.

Finally, it is useful to consider the role that alcohol plays in pathological aggression. Both the consumption of and the withdrawal from alcohol can contribute to pathological aggression (Helmy et al., 2020; Miczek et al., 2015; Vázquez-León et al., 2021). Individuals prone to use physical aggression and/

or to be reinforced primarily by the use of physical aggression tend to be more so under the influence of alcohol (Sontate et al., 2021). Similar links like those between alcohol and pathological aggression have not been established for other substances, like cocaine (Kuypers et al., 2020).

Conclusion

At the start of this chapter, we stated that reducing aggression may be the social goal the world most looks to psychology for helping accomplish. This is true both with reducing aggression exhibited by humans and also aggression exhibited by nonhuman animals (particularly those who live and work with humans). For these reasons, it seems appropriate to end this chapter with recommendations from comparative psychopathology and other psychological research for how to understand and possibly lessen aggression:

- It is important to remember that physical aggression is always an important part of social learning. There is no way to eliminate aggression and identifying problems requires understanding aggression on a continuum.
- Pathological aggression can be difficult to target because it is difficult to define. It is primarily thought of aggression that goes beyond what is needed for obtaining needed resources. That is difficult to define precisely because of variations in defining what is "needed" and also because it is hard to predict what will be "needed".
- Aggression is a primary factor in achieving social dominance but the process by which dominance occurs does not always involve physical aggression. Signaling that aggression could occur is most often the way that aggression maintains social dominance. Animals of a species tend to recognize and follow the social hierarchy rules that maintain a social hierarchy, even if no physical aggression occurs for its maintenance. This is why behaviors like threats and verbal aggression play so prominent a role in social networks.
- Social dominance maintained through signaling the possibility of physical aggression, with the associated possibilities of winning or losing social competitions, accounts both for aggressive and aggression-signaling behaviors in social group and depressive behaviors, signaling deference and surrender, in social groups. Interventions used to help lessen aggression and aggression-related behaviors for humans should focus on helping the individual re-interpret whether their interpretation that their social standing is in jeopardy or whether they are likely to lose the fight is rational and realistic. Interventions geared towards domesticating nonhuman animals should focus on withdrawing their interactions with social groups emphasizing dominance the animal is not likely to reach or maintain. These interventions should also focus on helping the animal learn they can

obtain needed resources regardless of how their dominance in a social group is interpreted.

- Social instigation (aggression triggered by social conflicts), social aggression (being reinforced for aggressive behaviors through social praise and attention) and social isolation (being left by oneself) are three of the main social stressors contributing to an overreliance on aggression. These are the types of social situations that interventions should target.

- Pathological aggression occurs when an aggressive behaviors become reinforcing in and of itself. An individual relies on physical aggression because the act itself becomes reinforcing. This is often because physical aggression is learned to be a part of so many types of situations (as part of it being a strong package of knowledge whose use is triggered in many situations where the behavior is reinforced) that it is more strongly reinforced as a behavior than would otherwise be the case.

- Interventions focused on lessening physical aggression should focus on those helping break the individual's knowledge pattern by helping them learn new skills that obtain the same type and level of reinforcement. These are approaches that should also focus on the individual's strengths and characteristics, rather than trying to change these basic aspects of the individual's self. Positive psychology interventions, seen through this perspective, are particularly helpful for addressing human aggression.

- Reinforcement schedules that tend to best address aggression are either fixed-ratio or fixed-interval schedules.

- Genetic predispositions for pathological aggression are likely to be the same ones associated with impulsivity.

- Interventions used to address pathological aggression in humans should also be ones that allow for also incorporating interventions for addressing pathological alcohol use.

References

Agbaria, Q. (2021). Internet addiction and aggression: The mediating roles of self-control and positive affect. *International Journal of Mental Health and Addiction, 19*(4), 1227–1242.

Albert, D. J., Walsh, M. L., & Jonik, R. H. (1993). Aggression in humans: What is its biological foundation? *Neuroscience & Biobehavioral Reviews, 17*(4), 405–425.

Arslan, G., Allen, K. A., & Tanhan, A. (2021). School bullying, mental health, and wellbeing in adolescents: Mediating impact of positive psychological orientations. *Child Indicators Research, 14*, 1007–1026.

Azevedo, J., Vieira-Coelho, M., Castelo-Branco, M., Coelho, R., & Figueiredo-Braga, M. (2020). Impulsive and premeditated aggression in male offenders with antisocial personality disorder. *PLoS One, 15*(3), e0229876.

Babcock, J. C., Tharp, A. L., Sharp, C., Heppner, W., & Stanford, M. S. (2014). Similarities and differences in impulsive/premeditated and reactive/proactive bimodal classifications of aggression. *Aggression and Violent Behavior, 19*(3), 251–262.

Bai, Q., Bai, S., Huang, Y., Hsueh, F. H., & Wang, P. (2020). Family incivility and cyberbullying in adolescence: A moderated mediation model. *Computers in Human Behavior, 110*, 106315.

Bandura, A., Ross, D., & Ross, S. A. (1963). Vicarious reinforcement and imitative learning. *The Journal of Abnormal and Social Psychology, 67*(6), 601–607. https://doi.org/10.1037/h0045550

Barratt, E. S., Stanford, M. S., Dowdy, L., Liebman, M. J., & Kent, T. A. (1999). Impulsive and premeditated aggression: a factor analysis of self-reported acts. *Psychiatry Research, 86*(2), 163–173.

Berkowitz, L. (1983). Aversively stimulated aggression: Some parallels and differences in research with animals and humans. *American Psychologist, 38*(11), 1135–1144. https://doi.org/10.1037/0003-066X.38.11.1135

Blanchard, D. C., & Blanchard, R. J. (2003). What can animal aggression research tell us about human aggression?. *Hormones and Behavior, 44*(3), 171–177.

Bushman, B. J., & Anderson, C. A. (2001). Is it time to pull the plug on hostile versus instrumental aggression dichotomy?. *Psychological Review, 108*(1), 273.

Coccaro, E. F. (2012). Intermittent explosive disorder as a disorder of impulsive aggression for DSM-5. *American Journal of Psychiatry, 169*(6), 577–588.

Coccaro, E. F., & Lee, R. J. (2020). Disordered aggression and violence in the United States. *The Journal of Clinical Psychiatry, 81*(2), 9267.

Coppens, C. M., de Boer, S. F., Buwalda, B., & Koolhaas, J. M. (2014). Aggression and aspects of impulsivity in wild-type rats. *Aggressive Behavior, 40*(4), 300–308.

Corsetti, S., Borruso, S., Malandrucco, L., Spallucci, V., Maragliano, L., Perino, R., Maragliano, L., Perino, R., D'Agostino, P. & Natoli, E. (2021). Cannabis sativa L. may reduce aggressive behaviour towards humans in shelter dogs. *Scientific Reports, 11*(1), 2773.

Couppis, M. H., & Kennedy, C. H. (2008). The rewarding effect of aggression is reduced by nucleus accumbens dopamine receptor antagonism in mice. *Psychopharmacology, 197*, 449–456.

Covington III, H. E., Newman, E. L., Leonard, M. Z., & Miczek, K. A. (2019). Translational models of adaptive and excessive fighting: an emerging role for neural circuits in pathological aggression. *F1000Research, 8*.

Cui, G., & Lan, X. (2020). The associations of parental harsh discipline, adolescents' gender, and grit profiles with aggressive behavior among Chinese early adolescents. *Frontiers in Psychology, 11*, 323.

de Almeida, R. M., & Miczek, K. A. (2002). Aggression escalated by social instigation or by discontinuation of reinforcement ("frustration") in mice: inhibition by anpirtoline: a 5-HT1B receptor agonist. *Neuropsychopharmacology, 27*(2), 171–181.

Eibl-Eibesfeldt, L. (1977). Evolution of destructive aggression. *Aggressive Behavior, 3*(2), 127–144.

Elwood, R. W., & Arnott, G. (2012). Understanding how animals fight with Lloyd Morgan's canon. *Animal Behaviour, 84*(5), 1095–1102.

Field, T. (2021). Aggression and violence affecting youth during the COVID-19 pandemic: A narrative review. *Journal of Psychiatry Research Reviews & Reports, 129*.

Fish, E. W., De Bold, J. F., & Miczek, K. A. (2002). Aggressive behavior as a reinforcer in mice: activation by allopregnanolone. *Psychopharmacology, 163*, 459–466.

Freud, A. (1947). Aggression in relation to emotional development; normal and pathological. *The Psychoanalytic Study of the Child, 3*(1), 37–42.

García-Vázquez, F. I., Valdés-Cuervo, A. A., & Parra-Pérez, L. G. (2020). The effects of forgiveness, gratitude, and self-control on reactive and proactive aggression in bullying. *International Journal of Environmental Research and Public Health*, *17*(16), 5760.

Garofalo, C., Neumann, C. S., & Velotti, P. (2021). Psychopathy and aggression: The role of emotion dysregulation. *Journal of Interpersonal Violence*, *36*(23–24), NP12640–NP12664.

Golden, S. A., Heins, C., Venniro, M., Caprioli, D., Zhang, M., Epstein, D. H., & Shaham, Y. (2017). Compulsive addiction-like aggressive behavior in mice. *Biological Psychiatry*, *82*(4), 239–248.

Greenebaum, J. B. (2010). Training dogs and training humans: Symbolic interaction and dog training. *Anthrozoös*, *23*(2), 129–141.

Haller, J. (2022). Aggression, aggression-related psychopathologies and their models. *Frontiers in Behavioral Neuroscience*, *16*, 936105.

Haller, J., & Kruk, M. R. (2006). Normal and abnormal aggression: Human disorders and novel laboratory models. *Neuroscience & Biobehavioral Reviews*, *30*(3), 292–303.

Harat, M., Rudaś, M., Zieliński, P., Birska, J., & Sokal, P. (2015). Deep brain stimulation in pathological aggression. *Stereotactic and Functional Neurosurgery*, *93*(5), 310–315.

Helmy, M., Zhang, J., & Wang, H. (2020). Neurobiology and neural circuits of aggression. *Neural Circuits of Innate Behaviors*, 9–22.

Hiday, V. A. (1995). The social context of mental illness and violence. *Journal of Health and Social Behavior*, 122–137.

Hobson, E. A. (2020). Differences in social information are critical to understanding aggressive behavior in animal dominance hierarchies. *Current Opinion in Psychology*, *33*, 209–215.

Hobson, E. A., Mønster, D., & DeDeo, S. (2021). Aggression heuristics underlie animal dominance hierarchies and provide evidence of group-level social information. *Proceedings of the National Academy of Sciences*, *118*(10), e2022912118.

Huesmann, L. R. (1998). The role of social information processing and cognitive schema in the acquisition and maintenance of habitual aggressive behavior. In: *Human Aggression* (pp. 73–109). Academic Press.

Huntingford, F. A., & Turner, A. K. (1987). *Animal Conflict*. Cambridge: Cambridge University Press.

Jacobs, C., De Keuster, T., & Simoens, P. (2003). Assessing the pathological extent of aggressive behaviour in dogs. A review of the literature. *Veterinary Quarterly*, *25*(2), 53–60.

Jager, A., Amiri, H., Bielczyk, N., van Heukelum, S., Heerschap, A., Aschrafi, A., & Glennon, J. C. (2020). Cortical control of aggression: GABA signalling in the anterior cingulate cortex. *European Neuropsychopharmacology*, *30*, 5–16.

Kohl, J., Autry, A. E., & Dulac, C. (2017). The neurobiology of parenting: A neural circuit perspective. *Bioessays*, *39*(1), 1–11.

Kuik, M. M. (2022). *The Addiction of Aggression-Why Aggressive Behavior can be seen as Addictive Behavior* (Doctoral dissertation).

Kuypers, K. P., Verkes, R. J., van den Brink, W., van Amsterdam, J. G., & Ramaekers, J. G. (2020). Intoxicated aggression: Do alcohol and stimulants cause dose-related aggression? A Review. *European Neuropsychopharmacology*, *30*, 114–147.

Lee, T. M. C., Chan, S. C., & Raine, A. (2008). Strong limbic and weak frontal activation to aggressive stimuli in spouse abusers. *Molecular Psychiatry*, *13*(7), 655–656.

Li, Y., & Dulac, C. (2018). Neural coding of sex-specific social information in the mouse brain. *Current Opinion in Neurobiology*, *53*, 120–130.

Lischinsky, J. E., & Lin, D. (2020). Neural mechanisms of aggression across species. *Nature Neuroscience*, *23*(11), 1317–1328.

Loew, C. A. (1967). Acquisition of a hostile attitude and its relationship to aggressive behavior. *Journal of Personality and Social Psychology*, *5*(3), 335–341. https://doi.org/10.1037/h0024259

May, M. E., & Kennedy, C. H. (2009). Aggression as positive reinforcement in mice under various ratio-and time-based reinforcement schedules. *Journal of the Experimental Analysis of Behavior*, *91*(2), 185–196.

Miczek, K. A., de Almeida, R. M., Kravitz, E. A., Rissman, E. F., de Boer, S. F., & Raine, A. (2007). Neurobiology of escalated aggression and violence. *Journal of Neuroscience*, *27*(44), 11803–11806.

Miczek, K. A., de Boer, S. F., & Haller, J. (2013). Excessive aggression as model of violence: a critical evaluation of current preclinical methods. *Psychopharmacology*, *226*, 445–458.

Miczek, K. A., Takahashi, A., Gobrogge, K. L., Hwa, L. S., & de Almeida, R. M. (2015). Escalated aggression in animal models: shedding new light on mesocorticolimbic circuits. *Current Opinion in Behavioral Sciences*, *3*, 90–95.

Mos, J., & Olivier, B. (1991). Concepts in animal models for pathological aggressive behaviour in humans. *Animal Models in Psychopharmacology*, 297–316.

Natarajan, D., & Caramaschi, D. (2010). Animal violence demystified. *Frontiers in Behavioral Neuroscience*, *4*, 887.

Onyike, C., & Lyketsos, C. (2011). Aggression and violence. *Textbook of Psychosomatic Medicine: Psychiatric Care of the Medically Ill*, *101*, 153–174.

Owens, R. L., & Waters, L. (2020). What does positive psychology tell us about early intervention and prevention with children and adolescents? A review of positive psychological interventions with young people. *The Journal of Positive Psychology*, *15*(5), 588–597.

Pisano, S., & Masi, G. (2020). Recommendations for the pharmacological management of irritability and aggression in conduct disorder patients. *Expert Opinion on Pharmacotherapy*, *21*(1), 5–7.

Pompili, E., Carlone, C., Silvestrini, C., & Nicolò, G. (2017). Focus on aggressive behaviour in mental illness. *Rivista di psichiatria*, *52*(5), 175–179.

Potegal, M. (1979). The reinforcing value of several types of aggressive behavior: A review. *Aggressive Behavior*, *5*(4), 353–373.

Price, E. O. (1999). Behavioral development in animals undergoing domestication. *Applied Animal Behaviour Science*, *65*(3), 245–271.

Prinzing, M. M. (2021). Positive psychology is value-laden—It's time to embrace it. *The Journal of Positive Psychology*, *16*(3), 289–297.

Prunier, A., Averos, X., Dimitrov, I., Edwards, S. A., Hillmann, E., Holinger, M., … & Camerlink, I. (2020). Early life predisposing factors for biting in pigs. *Animal*, *14*(3), 570–587.

Range, F., & Marshall-Pescini, S. (2022). Comparing wolves and dogs: Current status and implications for human 'self-domestication'. *Trends in Cognitive Sciences*.

Reite, M., Short, R., Kaufman, I., Stynes, A., & Pauley, J. (1978). Heart rate and body temperature in separated monkey infants. *Biological Psychiatry*, *73*, 91–105.

Resta, E., Kruglanski, A. W., Ellenberg, M., & Pierro, A. (2023). Ambition-driven aggression in response to significance-threatening frustration. *European Journal of Social Psychology*, *53*(7), 1458–1474.

Riemer, S., Heritier, C., Windschnurer, I., Pratsch, L., Arhant, C., & Affenzeller, N. (2021). A review on mitigating fear and aggression in dogs and cats in a veterinary setting. *Animals*, *11*(1), 158.

Shizuka, D. & McDonald, D. B. (2015). The network motif architecture of dominance hierarchies. *Journal of The Royal Society Interface*, *12*, 20150080–20150080. URL https://royalsocietypublishing.org/doi/full/10.1098/rsif.2015.0080.

Sluyter, F., Takahashi, A., & Maxson, S. C. (2014). Pathological aggression. *Behavioral Genetics of the Mouse: Volume 2, Genetic Mouse Models of Neurobehavioral Disorders*, 86.

Sontate, K. V., Rahim Kamaluddin, M., Naina Mohamed, I., Mohamed, R. M. P., Shaikh, M. F., Kamal, H., & Kumar, J. (2021). Alcohol, aggression, and violence: from public health to neuroscience. *Frontiers in Psychology*, *12*, 699726.

Suomi, S. J. (2005, July). Aggression and social behaviour in rhesus monkeys. In *Molecular Mechanisms Influencing Aggressive Behaviours: Novartis Foundation Symposium 268* (pp. 216–226). Chichester, UK: John Wiley & Sons, Ltd.

Takahashi, A. (2021). Social stress and aggression in murine models. In: K. A. Miczek & R. Sinha, (Eds.). *Neuroscience of Social Stress. Current Topics in Behavioral Neurosciences*, vol 54. Cham: Springer. https://doi.org/10.1007/7854_2021_243

Thompson, T. (1961). Effect of chloropromazine on "aggressive" responding in the rat. *Journal of Comparative and Physiological Psychology*, *54*(4), 398–400.

Thompson, T. (1966). Operant and classically-conditioned aggressive behavior in Siamese fighting fish. *American Zoologist*, *6*(4), 629–641.

Tibbetts, E. A., Pardo-Sanchez, J., & Weise, C. (2022). The establishment and maintenance of dominance hierarchies. *Philosophical Transactions of the Royal Society B*, *377*(1845), 20200450.

Van den Berg, L., Vos-Loohuis, M., Schilder, M. B. H., Van Oost, B. A., Hazewinkel, H. A. W., Wade, C. M. & Leegwater, P. A. J. (2008). Evaluation of the serotonergic genes htr1A, htr1B, htr2A, and slc6A4 in aggressive behavior of golden retriever dogs. *Behavior Genetics*, *38*, 55–66.

Van Heukelum, S., Tulva, K., Geers, F. E., van Dulm, S., Ruisch, I. H., Mill, J. & França, A. S. (2021). A central role for anterior cingulate cortex in the control of pathological aggression. *Current Biology*, *31*(11), 2321–2333.

Varshney, M., Mahapatra, A., Krishnan, V., Gupta, R., & Deb, K. S. (2015). Violence and mental illness: what is the true story?. *Journal of Epidemiology and Community Health*.

Vázquez-León, P., Miranda-Páez, A., Calvillo-Robledo, A., & Marichal-Cancino, B. A. (2021). Blockade of GPR55 in dorsal periaqueductal gray produces anxiety-like behaviors and evocates defensive aggressive responses in alcohol-pre-exposed rats. *Neuroscience Letters*, *764*, 136218.

Wagels, L., Habel, U., Raine, A., & Clemens, B. (2022). Neuroimaging, hormonal and genetic biomarkers for pathological aggression—success or failure?. *Current Opinion in Behavioral Sciences*, *43*, 101–110.

Wlodarczyk, J. (2017). Be more dog: The human–Canine relationship in contemporary dog-training methodologies. *Performance Research*, *22*(2), 40–47.

10 Deprivation-Induced Psychopathology

Introduction

In this final chapter, we look at the role of a major environmental factor impacting behavior and psychopathology that rarely gets considered completely on its own: deprivation. We refer here to deprivation, defined as the lack of material benefits deemed necessary for a society. Other definitions for deprivation include the *Cambridge Dictionary* definition of "an absence or too little of something considered important" (Cambridge University, 2024) and the *Oxford University Dictionary* definition of "the fact of not having something that you need" (Oxford University, 2024).

Although, as we will discuss in this chapter, deprivation serves a major role in psychopathology, we are either the first or one of the few authors to specifically use the term "deprivation-induced psychopathology." We see this term as important because it puts the focus directly on the role of deprivation in causing and maintaining psychopathology. Too often, in our opinion, the increased prevalence of psychological disorders associated with individuals, human and nonhuman animals alike, has a "blame the victim" approach. People with mental health problems are seen as psychologically weak, and this leads them to suffer poverty (Pak, 2020). Animals in zoos cannot adapt, so they develop pathological behaviors in captivity. Deprivation is seen as an outcome of the pathology rather than its root cause. In our opinion, the term "deprivation-induced psychopathology" puts the focus where it needs to be: deprivation as a cause and not an outcome.

Essential Place of Deprivation in Fully Understanding Psychopathology

As we look at deprivation as a root cause throughout this chapter, we will address several different forms. For nonhuman animals, this includes maternal deprivation (being separated early from maternal care), food deprivation (lack of access to food due to natural disasters or other environmental conditions), and social deprivation (lack of access to social interactions). Each of these has a major impact on psychopathology as exhibited through animal behaviors. Comparative psychology has had a particularly important place in considering this as it impacts nonhuman animals because of how it has led to not only an understanding of psychological constructs but also changes in zoos and laboratories.

Issues related to deprivation-induced psychopathology for nonhuman animals strongly impact humans as well. Lack of access to quality parental care, lack of access to adequate food and shelter, and social isolation all affect humans and contribute directly to psychopathology. But we will give particular focus here on one aspect of human society that is itself defined as deprivation and also incorporates all other aspects of deprivation: poverty.

Poverty is the lack of material resources needed to survive and thrive in human society. It is typically thought of as lacking money and, as a result, things money can buy (food, shelter, clothing). This is accurate, although poverty also impacts many other areas of human life. Lack of financial resources leads to living in neighborhoods where safety and security are more concerned. When humans live in poverty, getting things needed just to survive takes more time and effort, so parental time for children is more limited. Time restraints associated with living in poverty also lead to more social isolation. Healthy food and other things needed for healthy lifestyles are more expensive, so physical health is also impacted by humans living in poverty. In short, all areas of deprivation that can impact psychopathology do impact psychopathology impacted or caused by poverty.

Incorporating the issues of deprivation-induced and particularly poverty-induced pathology into the comparative psychopathology path of under-standing psychological disorders is a major strength. For most of psychology's history, poverty has not been adequately addressed. Professional and academic psychology has failed to address the concern of the poor and marginalized whose mental health difficulties have major contributions from external sources (Awaritefe, 2020; Bhattacharyya & Brenner, 2021; Krawitz & Watson, 1997; Madu, 2020; Ridley et al., 2020). This is undoubtedly true of all areas of psychology, but maybe the most obvious is the area of clinical psychology. This quote summarizes the problem well:

> "Nowhere is the futility of psychotherapy as obvious as among the poor and powerless whose suffering, crowding, and despair will yield only to social and political solutions"
>
> (Albee, 1990, p. 369).

Indeed, the difficulty here may rest in poverty being an external factor and psychology, particularly clinical psychology, which often focuses on internal factors (emotions, motivation, intelligence and the like). But the problem with much of psychology is that its focus on the internal and minimizing the external has worsened the problem. Clinical psychology has served a role in harming the emotional well-being of people living in poverty by pathologizing them (i.e., implying that mental health problems led to their poverty as opposed to their poverty leading to mental health problems) and creating barriers to care (Appio et al., 2013). Psychology as a profession and field of study has often been involved in widening the gap between advantaged and disadvantaged (or, in other terms, the difference between the "haves" and have nots"). This has mostly likely been inadvertent, but this does not change the fact that it needs to be addressed (Ceci & Papierno, 2005; Du & King, 2022; Guttentag, 1965; Jetten et al., 2020; Ordabayeva & Lisjak, 2022; Peters et al., 2022; Seidman, 1988).

Much of psychology's history has been focused on the "haves" over the "have nots." This was brought up in the previous Chapter 9, and comparative psychology's role in addressing this issue will be addressed here. When clinical psychology started, case studies were written, diagnoses created, and treatment approaches developed based on the psychological functioning of humans who had resources (primarily money but also power and connections). Wealthy patients received psychoanalytic services in the time of Freud and contemporaries (Bennett, 2011). One book that has become a significant training text for psychoanalysts over the years is the book *The Technique and Practice of Psychoanalysis*, written by Ralph Greenson, who was a psychoanalyst to the super-rich and super-famous (Kirsner, 2007). Later forms of therapy also focused on the psychological struggles of people who had access to resources while ignoring those of people who did not (Bartram & Stewart, 2019; Campbell & Selby-Nelson, 2020; Hill, 1996).

It is not just that clinical psychology treatment has been primarily directed toward people with resources that should cause concern. Patients receiving treatment are how professionals are trained and how practitioners develop treatment strategies. Psychology's history, with its emphasis on the sufferings of people with money, power, and status, has been one where the treatment and understanding of psychopathology have emphasized the suffering of humans with resources. Add to this the longstanding history of research psychology focusing heavily on studying humans with resources (college students who are much more likely to come from families with resources people with the time to volunteer for studies), and you have a limited but accurate picture of how psychology as a field, and particularly the study of psychological disorders and their treatment, has focused more on the needs and experiences of people at the top of the social hierarchy and much less on those towards the bottom.

Incorporating the study of deprivation and its direct impact on psychopathology creates an approach to understanding psychological disorder that gives equal weight to the experiences of the "have-nots" as to the "haves."

Questioning "What is the impact of having less or none of what is needed in a society?" is asked on equal grounds as "What is the impact of internal struggles when external needs are not a concern?". It also directly addresses the complex question of how much psychopathology psychology can really address. If the problems of many are primarily impacted by what they do not have (food, shelter, security, independence), what needs to be addressed outside of what the individual does? Looking at deprivation is as much a societal issue when it comes to psychopathology as it is an individual issue. In this way, comparative psychopathology does not make understanding psychopathology easier, but it does make it more complete.

Deprivation and the History of Comparative Psychopathology

As we addressed in Chapter 9 deprivation has been an important area since the first-time comparative psychopathology has been considered a field. When Howard Liddell started his behavior farm, his focus was expected to be on standard types of psychological experiments. Only when Liddell started identifying the impact of being in a restricted setting, his meaningful work began (Kirk & Ramsden, 2018). When studying how animals reacted to being the subjects of experiments and limited freedom, he contributed to some of the earliest and most meaningful studies of stress. His work showed what happened when freedom was taken away, and animals were deprived of their ability to engage in behaviors they instinctually thought necessary. Researchers from many fields and around the world came to see what could be learned from observing the intense and meaningful impact of being deprived not only of resources but of freedom (Freeman, 1985).

Although Liddell provides a long-term naturalistic environment for studying the impact of deprivation, he is probably not the most prominent name in deprivation studies. In the history of psychology, the most prominent name would most likely be another comparative psychology researcher, Harry Harlow. His studies, considered controversial in modern psychology, separated baby monkeys early from their mothers and peers (Harlow et al.,1966; Radetzki, 2018; Seay et al., 1962). In modern times, his studies may be seen as unnecessary, given how the general agreement in society that social isolation and maternal separation have pathological impacts. But Harlow's work was some of the first consistent work showing empirically what had been suspected but not proven for centuries. What Harlow showed conclusively was that maternal and social deprivation lead to increased rates of depressive behaviors (including pathological social withdrawal), increased aggression, decreased activity, and decreased eating.

Harow's studies provided many important findings and led to additional research on the issue of maternal deprivation. Animals in laboratories, zoos, and living on farms often experience some type of maternal deprivations.

This is usually because these settings lead to animals being separated from their mothers earlier than what would happen out in the wild. Maternal deprivation can also occur because restrictive environments may limit maternal behaviors. Repetitive behaviors like those discussed earlier in this book often happen because of this type of maternal deprivation. Problems with anger management also usually occur (Latham & Mason, 2008). Research after Harlow also showed that maternal behaviors leads to poor social learning in animals (Levy et al., 2003). Animals who do not start out with the support of a maternal figure and adequate social stimuli develop mood and behavior problems associated generally with psychopathology (e.g., depressive behaviors, repetitive behaviors, aggression).

Although Harlow's research and those that came after him contributed a great deal to the understanding of maternal deprivation, what is most important about his work on comparative psychopathology is what it contributed generally to pathology. Because Harlow's research was one of the first coordinated approaches to show that pathology occurs by the ABSENCE of something, it could be argued that up until that point, psychopathology had been seen as the result of SOMETHING happening to a person. Trauma, abuse, and violence were just some examples. Even the impact of dreams and upsetting memories were described as impacting a person's psychological functioning because they happened to the person. Melancholy, Freud's term for what would later be called clinical depression, emphasized mourning and loss (implying something missing that the person once had) rather than something never being there. Following the early days of psychoanalysis, cognitive therapists described pathology as resulting from irrational learning (an active process). Skinner, considered the founder of the behavioral school, implied absence to be the normal state of things when he described children as "blank slates" or "tabula rosa" (Pinker, 2003). In the major schools of psychological thought, absence was not emphasized as a major problem in psychological disorders.

Psychology's failure to address absence and deprivation as major issues led to a major gap not only in what it offered for individuals but also in what it offered to society. Much of the understanding of pathology and human development until psychology formalized as a science included the general idea that "people cannot be impacted by something they never had." Terrible things can happen to people and very often cause psychological distress. However, the idea that human and nonhuman animals could be impacted intensely and permanently by the absence of something was not emphasized. One could even argue that the works of Liddell and Harlow started and existed because the researchers themselves did not recognize until after analyzing their findings the impact of deprivation (both used animals who had freedom, social interactions, and maternal care removed either before individual animals were born or very soon after they were born). Again, the idea here is, "How can you be impacted by something you never knew you had?". This view not only impacted psychology but society as well. Rich had impacted the poor throughout history, justifying that their treatment of people experiencing poverty was not a problem since they had not done anything to them. Racism, sexism, and ableism all exist with the justification that the person does not really offend because they are not actually doing anything to the person (outside of the overt violence used to keep the offenses in place). Social ills have often existed with the idea that the individuals affected are not really being harmed by society if other individuals have not actually done anything to them but have just allowed deprivation to exist.

Considering the impact of deprivation fits into the benefit that comparative psychology has provided psychology throughout its history. When the research and other forms of academic knowledge related to animal behavior were used in psychology, they forced psychology to look at the darker side of human nature. This in no way meant that nonhuman animals were the only ones to display these darker aspects, but rather, studying animals allowed an experiential distance for considering these aspects until the time they could be applied to humans. As discussed earlier, Freud used the work of Darwin and his contemporaries to argue just how sexual and violent human animals could be even when they are developing normally. Jung then challenged Freud's theories by identifying that even the sexual and violent behaviors Freud had defined as deviant were actually quite natural when observing farm animals (which Jung had done for years growing up on a farm). Skinner's behavioral theories, based on his animal studies, showed that human and nonhuman animals very often seek their own individual rewards without any apparent consideration for others or motivation by intrinsic feelings and morals. Cognitive theories, which were an outgrowth of the behavioral approach, also emphasized focus on the self and individuals acting on their own view of the world (without necessarily being impacted by the opinions of others). The "cognitive revolution" in psychology (with its emphasis on individual motivation and perspectives) is considered a major contributor to the work of Ayn Rand and her objectivist philosophy focused on the benefits of individual happiness (Campbell, 1999). Harlow's work focused on how individuals and society in general harm other individuals not only by what is DONE to these individuals but also by what is NOT DONE for these individuals.

Harlow's work not only impacted the study of human and nonhuman animals but also led to real changes in how nonhuman animals were treated by humans. We are pleased to say that one of this book's authors (Maple) was instrumental in this change and was also strongly impacted by Harlow (Hoff et al., 1994; Maple, 2007, 2015; Maple et al., 1975; Maple & Finlay, 1989; Maple & Perdue, 2013; Ogden et al., 1990). His work impacted how animal laboratories functioned but even more dramatically impacted how zoos functioned. For decades, zoo animals were kept in cages with very limited room to move and very limited freedom to engage in what the animals felt natural. As discussed in this book's chapter on zoos, this led to several behaviors defined as pathological. Following the work of Harlow, with its focus on how depriving animals of something important (i.e., maternal care and social contact) could have the same degree of impact as doing something to the animal. Maple and colleagues worked not only through their academic publications but also in their professional capacities to make significant changes in how zoos operate. What zoo visitors see now in most zoos is a more naturalistic environment where animals have much more freedom to roam and interact with others than was the case decades ago. There is still much work to be done on zoos, and there is a robust debate on whether zoos should exist at all, but what exists now is much better for animals than what existed then.

Food Deprivation and Its Impact on Psychopathology

In the remainder of this chapter, we will look at samples of what psychological research, particularly comparative psychology research, offers to understand the impact of deprivation. These days, research is much more plentiful in addressing the effects of deprivation than it was years ago. What this chapter provides is just a small illustration of what the field of comparative psychopathology can offer in a more comprehensive view of both human and nonhuman psychological responses to deprivation. We have already addressed briefly the issue of maternal deprivation and will look next at the impact of food deprivation.

Studying food deprivation not only occurs in restricted environments like laboratories but also happens in ethology research. All animals face the possibility of food and resource limitations (McCue, 2010), and studying animals in their natural environments allows for studying how this impacts animal behavior. Food deprivation is associated with the behavioral state of starvation. In comparative psychology research, starvation refers to a condition where an animal who is otherwise willing or able to eat is unable to do so due to external limitations of food. How frequently this occurs and how prolonged starvation lasts varies widely. Weather events like tidal cycles or droughts are common causes of animal starvation.

Research on snails, crayfish, and certain crustations shows that animals tend to increase their behaviors initially when facing starvation but then decrease their activities (Alonso, 2021; Hazlett, 2003; Plath, 1998). When animals first face starvation, they will actively look for food, but when their searches are unsuccessful, they will slow down and be more limited in their search and activities. This behavioral response mirrors the biological changes associated with lacking nutrients and calories.

Interestingly, nonhuman animal research on starvation has shown behavioral similarities to the human psychological disorder of anorexia nervosa (Hebebrand et al., 2022). This is in part because anorexia involves self-starvation, which follows the same physiological path as starvation. One theory of anorexia is that it develops from significant difficulties leading to the person experiencing physiological responses indicating distress (Brockmeyer et al., 2012). What makes distressing emotional states different from anorexia compared to other types of distressing states is that the focus is primarily on body image and concerns about weight. In this way, the emotional distress triggers the same sort of physiological defenses associated with nonhuman animals who are starving (McCue, 2012). There is a particular focus on reducing caloric intake and reducing what would lead the body to need more calories (i.e., reducing body weight). Even the intense focus on exercise often associated with anorexia could be seen as similar but as a significant deviation from the starving animal's initial burst of activity when facing starvation.

Starvation, including starvation faced by nonhuman animals out in the wild and self-starvation faced by humans suffering from eating disorders, often triggers reactions to the social competition summarized in Chapter 3. This perspective helps account for the depressive behaviors exhibited by animals who are starving, and the high level of clinical depression associated with anorexia and other eating disorders (Laessle et al., 1988; Wilsdon & Wade, 2006). Intra-species competition determines which members of an animal group have access to limited food and resources (White, 2008). Facing starvation, whether caused by external events or self-imposed, leads to the physiological and cognitive responses associated with social competition. This leads to depression and other aspects of emotional distress, as being low on the social hierarchy has direct negative impacts on animals' stress levels and physical health (Sapolsky, 2004, 2005).

Food deprivation often leads to hoarding behaviors in animals. This may seem logical since the lack of food would lead to animals wanting to store food during and after experiencing times with no food. What is particularly interesting here is that over time or in particularly distressing situations involving starvation, or the fear of starvation, the hoarding behavior itself becomes rewarding, not the accumulation of food (Bohn, 2023; Buckley & Schneider, 2003; Morgan et al., 1943). In the same way that aggressive behaviors (as discussed in the chapter on aggression) can become rewarding in and of themselves, hoarding behaviors can function similarly.

Social Deprivation and Its Impact on Psychopathology

Lack of contact with others in an individual's social group is significantly associated with psychopathology. This occurs both through physiological and learning pathways. Social deprivation directly impacts behavioral and brain development associated with psychopathology (Humphreys et al.,

2017; Wadsworth et al., 2016). Deficits in social communication and effectively navigating social situations and relationships (i.e., social learning) are some of the main pathways by which deprivation leads to psychopathology in adolescence and young adulthood (Schafer et al., 2020).

When Harlow conducted his studies, the focus of his results was primarily on maternal contact and care deprivation (van Rosmalen et al., 2022). However, his studies also included the early and significant impact of having less contact with one's peers and social group. Social isolation increases the likelihood of psychopathology across the age spectrum (Baek, 2014). Research conducted during and after the COVID-19 pandemic emphasized the impact that social isolation has on psychopathology in all age groups (Rodman et al., 2021, 2022).

Comparative psychology research has shown the significance of social connection and social learning in how all animals develop and thrive. Being separated from one's social group leads to a lack of knowledge and a lack of connectedness that is genetically "hardwired" into all individuals. All individuals share a need to feel connected to others, even if different species have different needs for how much connection they need. Bears, for example, are some of the most individualized animals on earth. Even though they need less social interaction with peers than others, bears still need to feel socially connected. Throughout this book, we discussed how social hierarchies are maintained because of how individual members of a species recognize and acknowledge the hierarchy. This is just one example of the existence of a social connectedness need that exists beyond any need for learning or teaching. Animals need to feel socially connected in some way, and comparative psychology research shows a great deal of how that operates and what happens when it is removed.

Comparative psychology studies also show that the impact of social isolation can be reversed. What pathological impact social isolation has on animals' behaviors can be addressed by having individuals spend time around other members of their species. Social isolation often leads to more aggressive and individualistic behaviors, and increased social experiences and time in social settings can help to reverse this impact. In the research literature, one way this is applied is through a process called "urbanization," which involves being in settings where close contact with other members of a species is required. This approach tends to make animals more tolerant of each other and less likely to monopolize food and other resources (Cheney, 2011; Łopucki et al., 2021).

Poverty and Its Impact on Psychopathology

As stated earlier, poverty for humans represents the culmination of deprivation in all its forms. Poverty itself is deprivation, and other forms of deprivation (including social deprivation, freedom deprivation, emotional support deprivation, maternal deprivation, and food deprivation) are strongly associated with poverty. This explains why psychopathology is so strongly associated with poverty. Deprivation in childhood is significantly related to pathology in adolescence and early adulthood (McGoron et al., 2012; Miller et al., 2021; Milojevich et al., 2019; Schäfer et al., 2023). Poverty is often associated with deprivation of cognitive and social stimulation in infancy and early childhood, and this is one mechanism by which psychopathology in many forms develops (Sheridan & McLaughlin, 2014; Wadsworth, 2012). Low childhood socioeconomic status is associated with a significantly higher risk of lifelong psychopathology. This is primarily because of the amount of deprivation associated with poverty (Flouri et al., 2010; Ning et al., 2023; Weissman et al., 2022).

Children and teenagers from lower socioeconomic status and disadvantaged neighborhoods have a higher risk of psychopathology, primarily because of decreased access to rewards (Mullins et al., 2020). Research across the age spectrum shows that limited access to rewards significantly impacts the neurological pathways guiding how and why individuals seek rewards (Bjork et al., 2010; Hansen et al., 2016; Jenkins et al., 2020). Poverty has a significant impact on how human beings develop, and this leads to significant increases in psychological disorders. Depressive disorders occur more in people living in poverty (Galea et al., 2007; Kinyanda et al., 2011; Liao et al., 2023; Smith & Mazure, 2021); so do anxiety disorders (Ahulu et al., 2020; Alvand et al., 2020; Jiao et al., 2020), pathological gambling (Hahmann et al., 2021), and substance abuse disorders (Manhica et al., 2021).

Deprivation plays a significant role in the comparative psychopathology view of psychological disorders. Poverty impacts humans in many ways that lead to the development of psychopathology – viewing these disorders through the lens of comparative psychopathology demands that psychologists take more of an active role in understanding that human beings are impacted not by what society does to them but what society does not do for them. People living in poverty must be helped to recognize that their plight is not caused by something they did or that others did directly to them but by the impact of what was not done for them. Mental health professionals working with individuals living in poverty benefit their clients by helping them recognize that their socioeconomic condition that leads to their mental health problems more often than the other way around (Lawrence, 1982; Overholser, 2016; Sommet & Elliot, 2023).

This approach to understanding psychopathology also underscores the importance of psychology working outside of the therapy office or consulting room to address change that will truly impact certain types of psychopathologies. In the way that comparative psychologists like Maple and his colleagues used their understanding of deprivation-induced pathology to change the way that nonhuman animals were treated, it is important that psychologists, helped by the comparative psychopathology approach, work on a system level to address changes needed for helping humans suffering the impact of poverty and other types of deprivation. It is beyond the scope of this book to address specific steps on how this can be accomplished, but certainly one route would be the therapies that incorporate advocacy and political action into their approaches (Budge & Moradi, 2018; Grzanka & Miles, 2016; Richmond et al., 2013; Smith et al., 2013; Tone et al., 2022; Weiner, 2013; Zayas, 2001;).

Conclusion

We conclude our book with this chapter dedicated to one area in which comparative psychopathology has a unique role. Studying the direct impact of deprivation on pathological development has been a part of comparative psychology for much of its history. This field offers an understanding of how much of a major impact deprivation has on psychological development. Comparative psychology researchers have shown how much deprivation needs to be considered concerning nonhuman animals and why many suffer. Lack of food, shelter, safety, and water (among other resources) can be caused for many reasons in the wild, and lack of access to maternal care and freedom occurs for animals in captivity. Recognizing this moved forward psychology's understanding of nonhuman animals and what they need. It also led to changes in restrictive environments and how humans there treat nonhuman animals. In much the same way, a field of psychopathology study that incorporates comparative psychology research has the real opportunity to give much more importance to understanding the often devastating influence of deprivation, particularly with regard to poverty. We hope that what we provide here can be the start of comparative psychopathology having a major role in professional psychology, particularly its understanding of psychological disorders, for all who need help.

References

Ahulu, L. D., Gyasi-Gyamerah, A. A., & Anum, A. (2020). Predicting risk and protective factors of generalized anxiety disorder: a comparative study among adolescents in Ghana. *International Journal of Adolescence and Youth*, 25(1), 574–584.

Albee, G. W. (1990). The futility of psychotherapy. *The Journal of Mind and Behavior*, 369–384.

Alonso, Á. (2021). To eat or not to eat: the importance of starvation on behavioral bioassays. *Water, Air, & Soil Pollution*, 232, 1–9.

Alvand, S., Mohammadi, Z., Rashidian, L., Cheraghian, B., Rahimi, Z., Danehchin, L. & Poustchi, H. (2020). Irritable bowel syndrome: psychological disorder or poverty? Results of a large cross-sectional study in Iran. *Archives of Iranian medicine*, 23(12), 821–826.

Appio, L., Chambers, D. A., & Mao, S. (2013). Listening to the voices of the poor and disrupting the silence about class issues in psychotherapy. *Journal of Clinical Psychology, 69*(2), 152–161.

Awaritefe, A. (2020). Psychotherapy in Nigeria. *International Journal for Psychotherapy in Africa, 2*(1), 7–19.

Baek, S. B. (2014). Psychopathology of social isolation. *Journal of Exercise Rehabilitation, 10*(3), 143.

Bartram, M., & Stewart, J. M. (2019). Income-based inequities in access to psychotherapy and other mental health services in Canada and Australia. *Health policy, 123*(1), 45–50.

Bennett, D. (2011). 'Money is laughing gas to me'(Freud): a critique of pure reason in economics and psychoanalysis. *New Formations, 72*(72), 5–19.

Bhattacharyya, S., & Brenner, C. (2021). "Mending broken pieces": A group healing arts psychotherapy model. *Group, 45*(1), 31–52.

Bjork, J. M., Chen, G., Smith, A. R., & Hommer, D. W. (2010). Incentive-elicited mesolimbic activation and externalizing symptomatology in adolescents. *Journal of Child Psychology and Psychiatry, 51*(7), 827–837.

Bohn, S. (2023). *The Effects of Individual and Environmental Variation on a Food Hoarding Rodent's Stored Resources* (Doctoral dissertation, University of Guelph).

Brockmeyer, T., Holtforth, M. G., Bents, H., Kämmerer, A., Herzog, W., & Friederich, H. C. (2012). Starvation and emotion regulation in anorexia nervosa. *Comprehensive psychiatry, 53*(5), 496–501.

Buckley, C. A., & Schneider, J. E. (2003). Food hoarding is increased by food deprivation and decreased by leptin treatment in Syrian hamsters. *American Journal of Physiology-Regulatory, Integrative and Comparative Physiology, 285*(5), R1021–R1029.

Budge, S. L., & Moradi, B. (2018). Attending to gender in psychotherapy: Understanding and incorporating systems of power. *Journal of Clinical Psychology, 74*(11), 2014–2027.

Cambridge University (2024). Deprivation. Cambridge University Press, Cambridge Dictionary. https://dictionary.cambridge.org/dictionary/english/deprivation

Campbell, L. F., & Selby-Nelson, E. M. (2020). Bringing psychotherapy to people living in poverty. *Bringing Psychotherapy to the Underserved: Challenges and Strategies,* 98–122.

Campbell, R. L. (1999). Ayn Rand and the cognitive revolution in psychology. *The Journal of Ayn Rand Studies,* 107–134.

Ceci, S. J., & Papierno, P. B. (2005). The Rhetoric and Reality of Gap Closing: *When the "Have-Nots" Gain but the "Haves" Gain Even More. American Psychologist, 60*(2), 149–160. https://doi.org/10.1037/0003-066X.60.2.149

Cheney, D. L. (2011). Extent and limits of cooperation in animals. *Proceedings of the National Academy of Sciences, 108*(supplement_2), 10902–10909

Du, H., & King, R. B. (2022). The psychology of economic inequality and social class. *Asian Journal of Social Psychology, 25*(1), 3–6.

Flouri, E., Mavroveli, S., & Tzavidis, N. (2010). Modeling risks: Effects of area deprivation, family socio-economic disadvantage and adverse life events on young children's psychopathology. *Social Psychiatry and Psychiatric Epidemiology, 45,* 611–619.

Freeman, F. S. (1985). A reflection: Howard Scott Liddell, 1895–1962. *Journal of the History of the Behavioral Sciences, 21*(4), 372–374.

Galea, S., Ahern, J., Nandi, A., Tracy, M., Beard, J., & Vlahov, D. (2007). Urban neighborhood poverty and the incidence of depression in a population-based cohort study. *Annals of Epidemiology, 17*(3), 171–179.

Grzanka, P. R., & Miles, J. R. (2016). The problem with the phrase "intersecting identities": LGBT affirmative therapy, intersectionality, and neoliberalism. *Sexuality Research and Social Policy, 13*(4), 371–389.

Guttentag, M. (1965). A newcomer looks at school psychology: The problem of the "have-nots" in Suburbia. *Journal of School Psychology, 3*(4), 6–11.

Hahmann, T., Hamilton-Wright, S., Ziegler, C., & Matheson, F. I. (2021). Problem gambling within the context of poverty: A scoping review. *International Gambling Studies, 21*(2), 183–219.

Hanson, J. L., Albert, D., Iselin, A. M. R., Carre, J. M., Dodge, K. A., & Hariri, A. R. (2016). Cumulative stress in childhood is associated with blunted reward-related brain activity in adulthood. *Social Cognitive and Affective Neuroscience, 11*(3), 405–412.

Harlow, H. F., Harlow, M. K., Dodsworth, R. O., & Arling, G. L. (1966). Maternal behavior of rhesus monkeys deprived of mothering and peer associations in infancy. *Proceedings of the American Philosophical Society, 110*(1), 58–66.

Hazlett, B. A. (2003). The effects of starvation on crayfish responses to alarm odor. *Ethology, 109*(7), 587–592.

Hebebrand, J., Hildebrandt, T., Schlögl, H., Seitz, J., Denecke, S., Vieira, D. & Fulton, S. (2022). The role of hypoleptinemia in the psychological and behavioral adaptation to starvation: Implications for anorexia nervosa. *Neuroscience & Biobehavioral Reviews, 141*, 104807.

Hill, M. (1996). We can't afford it: Confusions and silences on the topic of class. *Women & Therapy, 18*(3–4), 1–5.

Hoff, M. P., Nadler, R. D., Hoff, K. T., & Maple, T. L. (1994). Separation and depression in infant gorillas. *Developmental Psychobiology: The Journal of the International Society for Developmental Psychobiology, 27*(7), 439–452.

Humphreys, K. L., Fox, N. A., Nelson, C. A., & Zeanah, C. H. (2017). Psychopathology following severe deprivation: History, research, and implications of the Bucharest Early Intervention Project. *Child Maltreatment in Residential Care: History, Research, and Current Practice*, 129–148.

Jenkins, L. M., Chiang, J. J., Vause, K., Hoffer, L., Alpert, K., Parrish, T. B. & Miller, G. E. (2020). Subcortical structural variations associated with low socioeconomic status in adolescents. *Human Brain Mapping, 41*(1), 162–171.

Jetten, J., Mols, F., & Selvanathan, H. P. (2020). How economic inequality fuels the rise and persistence of the Yellow Vest movement. *International Review of Social Psychology*, 33, 2. https://doi.org/10.5334/irsp.356

Jiao, C., Leng, A., Nicholas, S., Maitland, E., Wang, J., Zhao, Q. & Gong, C. (2020). Multimorbidity and mental health: the role of gender among disease-causing poverty, rural, aged households in China. *International Journal of Environmental Research and Public Health, 17*(23), 8855.

Kinyanda, E., Woodburn, P., Tugumisirize, J., Kagugube, J., Ndyanabangi, S., & Patel, V. (2011). Poverty, life events and the risk for depression in Uganda. *Social Psychiatry and Psychiatric Epidemiology, 46*, 35–44.

Kirk, R. G., & Ramsden, E. (2018). Working across species down on the farm: Howard S. Liddell and the development of comparative psychopathology, c. 1923–1962. *History and Philosophy of the Life Sciences, 40*, 1–29.

Kirsner, D. (2007). "Do as I say, not as I do": Ralph Greenson, Anna Freud, and superrich patients. *Psychoanalytic Psychology, 24*(3), 475–486.

Krawitz, R., & Watson, C. (1997). Gender, race and poverty: Bringing the sociopolitical into psychotherapy. *Australian & New Zealand Journal of Psychiatry, 31*(4), 474–479.

Laessle, R. G., Schweiger, U., & Pirke, K. M. (1988). Depression as a correlate of starvation in patients with eating disorders. *Biological Psychiatry, 23*(7), 719–725.

Latham, N. R., & Mason, G. J. (2008). Maternal deprivation and the development of stereotypic behaviour. *Applied Animal Behaviour Science, 110*(1–2), 84–108.

Lawrence, M. M. (1982). Psychoanalytic psychotherapy among poverty populations and the therapist's use of the self. *Journal of the American Academy of Psychoanalysis, 10*(2), 241–255.

Lévy, F., Melo, A. I., Galef Jr, B. G., Madden, M., & Fleming, A. S. (2003). Complete maternal deprivation affects social, but not spatial, learning in adult rats. *Developmental Psychobiology: The Journal of the International Society for Developmental Psychobiology, 43*(3), 177–191.

Liao, Y. A., Garcia-Mondragon, L., Konac, D., Liu, X., Ing, A., Goldblatt, R. & Barker, E. D. (2023). Nighttime lights, urban features, household poverty, depression, and obesity. *Current Psychology, 42*(18), 15453–15464.

Łopucki, R., Klich, D., & Kiersztyn, A. (2021). Changes in the social behavior of urban animals: more aggression or tolerance?. *Mammalian Biology, 101*, 1–10.

Madu, S. N. (2020). Psychotherapy training in Nigeria. *International Journal for Psychotherapy in Africa, 1*(1), 7–13.

Manhica, H., Straatmann, V. S., Lundin, A., Agardh, E., & Danielsson, A. K. (2021). Association between poverty exposure during childhood and adolescence, and drug use disorders and drug-related crimes later in life. *Addiction, 116*(7), 1747–1756.

Maple, T., Brandt, E. M., & Mitchell, G. (1975). Separation of preadolescents from infant rhesus monkeys. *Primates, 16*(2), 141–153.

Maple, T. L. (2007). Toward a science of welfare for animals in the zoo. *Journal of Applied Animal Welfare Science, 10*(1), 63–70.

Maple, T. L. (2015). Four decades of psychological research on zoo animal welfare. *Markus Gusset1 & Gerald Dick2, 24*, 41.

Maple, T. L., & Finlay, T. W. (1989). Applied primatology in the modern zoo. *Zoo Biology, 8*(S1), 101–116.

Maple, T. L., & Perdue, B. M. (2013). *Zoo Animal Welfare* (Vol. 14). Berlin, Germany: Springer.

McCue, M. D. (2010). Starvation physiology: reviewing the different strategies animals use to survive a common challenge. *Comparative Biochemistry and Physiology Part A: Molecular & Integrative Physiology, 156*(1), 1–18.

McCue, M. D. (2012). *Comparative physiology of fasting, starvation, and food limitation* (pp. 103–131). New York: Springer.

McGoron, L., Gleason, M. M., Smyke, A. T., Drury, S. S., Nelson III, C. A., Gregas, M. C., ... & Zeanah, C. H. (2012). Recovering from early deprivation: attachment mediates effects of caregiving on psychopathology. *Journal of the American Academy of Child & Adolescent Psychiatry, 51*(7), 683–693.

Miller, A. B., Machlin, L., McLaughlin, K. A., & Sheridan, M. A. (2021). Deprivation and psychopathology in the Fragile Families Study: A 15-year longitudinal investigation. *Journal of Child Psychology and Psychiatry, 62*(4), 382–391.

Milojevich, H. M., Norwalk, K. E., & Sheridan, M. A. (2019). Deprivation and threat, emotion dysregulation, and psychopathology: Concurrent and longitudinal associations. *Development and Psychopathology, 31*(3), 847–857.

Morgan, C. T., Stellar, E., & Johnson, O. (1943). Food–deprivation and hoarding in rats. *Journal of Comparative Psychology, 35*(3), 275–295. https://doi.org/10.1037/h0056707

Mullins, T. S., Campbell, E. M., & Hogeveen, J. (2020). Neighborhood deprivation shapes motivational–neurocircuit recruitment in children. *Psychological Science, 31*(7), 881–889.

Ning, K., Gondek, D., Pereira, S. M. P., & Lacey, R. E. (2023). Mediating mechanisms of the relationship between exposure to deprivation and threat during childhood and adolescent psychopathology: evidence from the Millennium Cohort Study. *European Child & Adolescent Psychiatry*, 1–14.

Ogden, J. J., Finlay, T. W., & Maple, T. L. (1990). Gorilla adaptations to naturalistic environments. *Zoo Biology, 9*(2), 107–121.

Ordabayeva, N., & Lisjak, M. (2022). Perceiving, coping with, and changing economic inequality in the marketplace. *Journal of Consumer Psychology, 32*(1), 165–174.

Overholser, J. C. (2016). When words are not enough: Psychotherapy with clients who are living below the poverty level. *Journal of Contemporary Psychotherapy, 46*, 89–96.

Oxford University (2024). *Deprivation.* Oxford University Press.

Pak, T. Y. (2020). Welfare stigma as a risk factor for major depressive disorder: evidence from the Supplemental Nutrition Assistance Program. *Journal of Affective Disorders, 260*, 53–60.

Peters, K., Jetten, J., Tanjitpiyanond, P., Wang, Z., Mols, F., & Verkuyten, M. (2022). The language of inequality: Evidence economic inequality increases wealth category salience. *Personality and Social Psychology Bulletin, 48*(8), 1204–1219.

Pinker, S. (2003). *The Blank Slate: The Modern Denial of Human Nature.* Penguin.

Plath, K. (1998). Adaptive feeding behavior of Duphnia magna in response to short-term starvation. *Limnology and Oceanography, 43*(4), 593–599.

Radetzki, P. (2018). Harlow's famous monkey study: The historical and contemporary significance of the nature of love. *Canadian Journal of Family and Youth/Le Journal Canadien de Famille et de la Jeunesse, 10*(1), 205–234.

Richmond, K., Geiger, E., & Reed, C. (2013). The personal is political: A feminist and trauma-informed therapeutic approach to working with a survivor of sexual assault. *Clinical Case Studies, 12*(6), 443–456.

Ridley, M., Rao, G., Schilbach, F., & Patel, V. (2020). Poverty, depression, and anxiety: Causal evidence and mechanisms. *Science, 370*(6522), eaay0214.

Rodman, A. M., Rosen, M. L., Kasparek, S. W., Mayes, M., Lengua, L., McLaughlin, K. A., & Meltzoff, A. N. (2021). *Social behavior and youth psychopathology during the COVID-19 pandemic: A longitudinal study.*

Rodman, A. M., Rosen, M. L., Kasparek, S. W., Mayes, M., Lengua, L., Meltzoff, A. N., & McLaughlin, K. A. (2022). Social experiences and youth psychopathology during the COVID-19 pandemic: A longitudinal study. *Development and Psychopathology*, 1–13.

Sapolsky, R. M. (2004). Social status and health in humans and other animals. *Annual Review of Anthropology, 33*, 393–418.

Sapolsky, R. M. (2005). The influence of social hierarchy on primate health. *Science, 308*(5722), 648–652.

Schäfer, J. L., McLaughlin, K. A., Manfro, G. G., Pan, P., Rohde, L. A., Miguel, E. C., & Salum, G. A. (2020). Cross-sectional and longitudinal associations of threat and deprivation on cognition, emotional processing and psychopathology in children and adolescents. *BioRxiv*, 2020-02.

Schäfer, J. L., McLaughlin, K. A., Manfro, G. G., Pan, P., Rohde, L. A., Miguel, E. C. & Salum, G. A. (2023). Threat and deprivation are associated with distinct aspects of cognition, emotional processing, and psychopathology in children and adolescents. *Developmental Science, 26*(1), e13267.

Seay, B., Hansen, E., & Harlow, H. F. (1962). Mother-infant separation in monkeys. *Journal of Child Psychology and Psychiatry, 3*(3-4), 123–132.

Seidman, E. (1988). Back to the future, community psychology: Unfolding a theory of social intervention. *American Journal of Community Psychology, 16*(1), 3–24.

Sheridan, M. A., & McLaughlin, K. A. (2014). Dimensions of early experience and neural development: deprivation and threat. *Trends in Cognitive Sciences, 18*(11), 580–585.

Smith, L., Li, V., Dykema, S., Hamlet, D., & Shellman, A. (2013). "Honoring somebody that society doesn't honor": Therapists working in the context of poverty. *Journal of Clinical Psychology, 69*(2), 138–151.

Smith, M. V., & Mazure, C. M. (2021). Mental health and wealth: Depression, gender, poverty, and parenting. *Annual Review of Clinical Psychology, 17*, 181–205.

Sommet, N., & Elliot, A. J. (2023). A competitiveness-based theoretical framework on the psychology of income inequality. *Current Directions in Psychological Science*, 09637214231159563.

Tone, J., Chelius, B., & Miller, Y. D. (2022). The effectiveness of a feminist-informed, individualised counselling intervention for the treatment of eating disorders: a case series study. *Journal of Eating Disorders, 10*(1), 1–12.

van Rosmalen, L., Luijk, M. P., & van der Horst, F. C. (2022). Harry Harlow's pit of despair: Depression in monkeys and men. *Journal of the History of the Behavioral Sciences, 58*(2), 204–222.

Wadsworth, M. E. (2012). Working with low-income families: Lessons learned from basic and applied research on coping with poverty-related stress. *Journal of Contemporary Psychotherapy, 42*, 17–25.

Wadsworth, M. E., Evans, G. W., Grant, K., Carter, J. S., & Duffy, S. (2016). Poverty and the development of psychopathology. *Developmental Psychopathology*, 1–44.

Weiner, K. M. (2013). Tools for change: Methods of incorporating political/social action into the therapy session. In Marcia Hill (Ed.), *Feminist Therapy as a Political Act* (pp. 113–123). Routledge.

Weissman, D. G., Rosen, M. L., Colich, N. L., Sambrook, K. A., Lengua, L. J., Sheridan, M. A., & McLaughlin, K. A. (2022). Exposure to violence as an environmental pathway linking low socioeconomic status with altered neural processing of threat and adolescent psychopathology. *Journal of Cognitive Neuroscience, 34*(10), 1892–1905.

White, T. (2008). The role of food, weather and climate in limiting the abundance of animals. *Biological Reviews, 83*(3), 227–248.

Wilsdon, A., & Wade, T. D. (2006). Executive functioning in anorexia nervosa: exploration of the role of obsessionality, depression and starvation. *Journal of Psychiatric Research, 40*(8), 746–754.

Zayas, L. H. (2001). Incorporating struggles with racism and ethnic identity in therapy with adolescents. *Clinical Social Work Journal, 29*, 361–373.

Index